A Special Report

How to Turn a Healthcare Crisis Into a Health Care Opportunity

What Can Happen
When Hospitals and Churches
Focus on Their Common Mission

STEPHANIE LIND, MBA &
SUSAN K. CHASE, EdD, RN, FNP-BC

FLORIDA HOSPITAL
Since 1908

FLORIDA
HOSPITAL

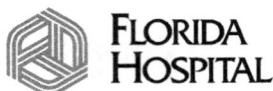

HOW TO TURN A HEALTHCARE CRISIS INTO
A HEALTH CARE OPPORTUNITY

Copyright © 2014 Florida Hospital Publishing
Published by Florida Hospital Publishing
900 Winderley Place, Suite 1600, Maitland, FL 32751

TO EXTEND *the* HEALING MINISTRY *of* CHRIST

EDITOR-IN-CHIEF	Todd Chobotar
MANAGING EDITOR	David Biebel, DMin
WRITER	Rainey Turlington
PRODUCTION	Lillian Boyd
COPY EDITOR	Pam Nordberg
PHOTOGRAPHY	Spencer Freeman
COVER DESIGN	Dana Boyd
INTERIOR DESIGN	The Herman Lewis Design Syndicate, LLC

PUBLISHER'S NOTE: This report is not intended to replace a one-on-one relationship with a qualified healthcare professional, but as a sharing of knowledge and information from the research and experience of the author. You are advised and encouraged to consult with your healthcare professional in all matters relating to your health and the health of your family. The publisher and authors disclaim any liability arising directly or indirectly from the use of this book.

AUTHORS' NOTE: This report contains many case histories and patient stories. In order to preserve the privacy of some of the people involved, we have disguised names, appearances, and aspects of their personal stories so they are not identifiable. Patient stories may also include composite characters.

For volume discounts please contact special sales at:
HealthProducts@FLHosp.org | 407-303-1929

Printed in the United States of America.
PR 15 14 13 12 11 10 9 8 7 6 5 4 3 2 1
ISBN 13: 978-0-9904191-1-2

For more life changing resources please visit:

FloridaHospitalPublishing.com

CreationHealth.com

Healthy100.org

CONTENTS

EDITOR'S INTRODUCTION

Today we are in a healthcare crisis. All around the industrialized world people are struggling with declining health. From childhood obesity to the multiple health-related needs and concerns of an aging population, millions need help understanding, managing, or even reversing their maladies. Hospitals are essential, of course, but most are set up for episodic care, not long-term disease management or continuous health improvement. So healthcare organizations, civic leaders, church leaders, and philanthropic groups wonder what can be done to help.

In this timely publication, authors Stephanie Lind of Florida Hospital and Dr. Susan Chase of the University of Central Florida share important insights and ideas based on a three-year pilot project involving Faith Community Nurses. Conducted in five Central Florida churches, the pilot sought to help congregations establish or grow an existing health ministry team. The work was accomplished through a partnership between Florida Hospital and the Winter Park Health Foundation. In these pages you'll discover the project goals, the methodology and processes used, and how others can take what was learned and do something similar—or better.

Pastors, church boards, Faith Community Nurses, hospitals, and many other concerned individuals – as well as organizations – can benefit from the lessons learned and documented in these pages. Lind and Chase have included many of the tools they used in the project that you may want to use or build on for future work.

Since this publication is written as more of a practical guide on how the study was conducted and how others can use the takeaways the authors learned, a second paper is planned by Chase and Lind that will present a detailed report and analysis of the project data. The second paper is intended for a professional audience and will be published in a peer-reviewed journal. As you read this, the second publication may already be available.

You may wonder why Florida Hospital – the largest admitting hospital in the United States – is involved in Faith Community Nursing and in helping churches start health ministries in their congregations. The answer is simple. For more than 100 years, the mission of Florida Hospital has been to extend the healing ministry of Christ. One of the ways the hospital fulfills this mission is by making individuals aware of the concepts of whole-person health and by assisting institutions such as churches (and businesses) learn how they can promote healthier living. In pursuit of this, Florida Hospital has a dedicated team of employees who work with churches to start, foster, and grow health ministries.

The project described in this report was one among many of Florida Hospital's ongoing efforts to help people understand how practicing the fundamentals of whole-person health aids in the prevention of disease and in recovery following an illness. I believe the authors have done a remarkable job of demonstrating how hospitals, churches, and Faith Community Nurses can positively affect the health of entire communities, playing a part in transforming our healthcare crisis into a health-caring opportunity. Worldwide health trends being what they are, that in itself is no small miracle.

Todd Chobotar
Publisher & Editor-in-Chief
Florida Hospital Publishing

PART 1

HEALTHCARE HAZARDS:
A CRISIS IN SEARCH OF A SOLUTION

In today's U.S. healthcare system, there is no single person whom a patient can count on to know and care about his or her mental, physical, and spiritual health.

A PREVENTABLE MISTAKE

It is only her first day home from the hospital and already Meredith feels exhausted and discouraged. At seventy-four years old, she knows she isn't a spring chicken, but at least before the surgery she could move around easily enough to do chores and enjoy her garden. Now, forced to use a walker for at least three months while her hip recovers, she struggles just to get out of bed. She decides to pass up a shower since she is so unsteady on her feet, and hobbles instead to the kitchen to cook breakfast.

Upon opening the refrigerator, Meredith sees that she has three eggs left, a little milk, some stale bread, a variety of partially used jams and jellies, and some dill pickles. Since she lives alone, there has been no one to purchase groceries while she was at the rehabilitation facility following her hip surgery, and before her admission she was in too much pain to go shopping. She closes the door with a sigh and looks wistfully at the pictures of her children and grandchildren stuck with magnets to the refrigerator door. They had called to see how she was doing, but none could get off work to spend a few weeks with her during her recovery.

Instead of frying up an egg, Meredith pulls open the drawer that holds her prescription medications. She sits down at the table to examine the new one her orthopedic surgeon has just prescribed for her. Squinting, she tries to make sense of the label and to recall his instructions, but her memory is as foggy this morning as it was when she first came out from under the influence of the anesthesia.

Rx 1: One Celecoxib 100 mg with food in the morning and evening.
Rx 2: One Rivaroxaban 10 mg daily for 35 days.
Rx 3: Percocet, one morning, one evening.
Rx 4: One Levofloxacin without food in the morning.
Rx 5: OxyContin—this is the new one. One 10 mg tablet in the morning for post-operative pain.

"I certainly have a lot of that today," she says to no one in particular as she places that tablet alongside the others she is about to ingest.

She feels like a human pharmacy for a moment. What she doesn't realize is that her surgeon has prescribed one of the same medications that she is already taking, as prescribed by her primary care physician, whose office is not affiliated with the surgeon's hospital. The hospital pharmacy has filled the surgeon's script and sent it home with her. Meredith says a prayer that she has remembered the instructions correctly as she gulps the pills down with water.

An hour-and-a-half later, Meredith arrives at church, thankful that another member was willing to pick her up. She shuffles in through the front door and past the cheerful greeters, her eyes fixed on a chair in the lobby where she knows she can stop to catch her breath. Apart from her time in the hospital, Meredith has not missed a single church service for the past fifteen years, and she doesn't want to miss one now. After a few minutes of rest, she painfully pulls herself back up from the chair and proceeds inside the sanctuary, where she takes a seat in the pew next to you. You are a member of the church's outreach committee, and you had heard that Meredith was home from surgery.

"Hello, Meredith," you whisper, touching her hand lightly. "How are you? I heard the surgery went well, and I was planning to come by tomorrow."

"Good," she replies. "I'm not having so much pain right now, but I feel so tired...." Then she nods, and it takes you a moment to realize that she has actually nodded off to sleep.

"Meredith," you whisper into her ear, but she just murmurs something. You catch the eye of an usher and make it clear that you need his help. Meredith wakes enough to seat herself in the wheelchair provided by the usher. You and he escort her out to the foyer, where she mumbles something about her meds. You realize that she needs a ride home immediately and someone to stay with her for at least a few hours until her situation improves, or if not, to get her back to the hospital. You wish there was a better way to offer help.

TOWARD A WHOLISTIC SOLUTION

In our current model of healthcare, talented medical professionals are trapped in a system where the majority of profits are made by completing procedures such as diagnostic tests and surgeries rather than providing health education or attempting to prevent diseases.

In this system, if an elderly gentleman is experiencing severe knee pain, it is likely that his physician will advise him to have surgery. While the two may discuss some of the pros and cons of the procedure, there are many other areas related to the patient's health that may not come up. These include whether or not he is emotionally prepared to deal with the stress of the operation, or if there is enough support at home to help care for him after the procedure. Depending on the physician, it could also include a discussion of alternative treatments and the different effects they can have on quality of life. Investigative reports have claimed that many procedures like this are unnecessary, or have limited benefit to the patient, yet the number of them taking place grows each year.[1] In other words, what we have is not a proactive healthcare system; it is a responsive disease management system.

Because the current model is not designed to support people having healthy, enriched lives that are within their control, millions suffer with chronic diseases such as diabetes, depression, cancer, heart disease, hypertension, and asthma. Many of these chronic conditions are related to the pandemic of obesity in our nation, afflicting old and young alike. According to the Centers for Disease Control and Prevention, "chronic diseases are among the most common, costly, and preventable of all health problems in the U.S." – accounting for 75 percent of healthcare costs in the United States and 60 percent of all deaths globally.[2] Through education and lifestyle changes, they are avoidable, but that is not what medical providers are paid to provide.

Compounding the problem is the fact that most medical offices are set up to address different specialty areas rather than provide whole-person care. They each do a good job in their own way, but no one is putting all of the pieces of the puzzle together. For example, an orthopedic surgeon can complete a successful surgery with clean incisions but afterward may be focused on helping the patient manage pain, unintentionally overlooking the fact that certain medications, or combinations of medications, that accomplish that purpose can also make an older person confused, as in the case of Meredith. Medication mix-up and resulting overdose is a growing cause of complications or death among older Americans.[3] A major contributor to this problem is that older Americans (age 65+) average about thirty prescriptions a year, with the highest average being 40.4 prescriptions per year by older residents of Kentucky.[4]

Even if patients receive excellent instructions in the hospital or doctor's office, they may not remember them all. Or, once at home, they may get confused. The list of things that could go wrong can become quite long, including communication errors and missed appointments.

Again, physicians are not usually trained or funded to develop a plan of care that addresses the person's full range of health issues – mental, physical, and spiritual. Although systems do exist to enable a patient's caregivers to communicate with one another to create a congruent treatment plan, the reality is that this rarely happens.

In today's U.S. healthcare system, there is no single person whom a patient can count on to know and care about his or her mental, physical, and spiritual health. However, Faith Community Nurses can do this. They can help patients reconcile their list of medications, serve as a health educator, provide ongoing health assessments in between appointments, and also minister to other needs that may arise.

Another example: A woman who has just been diagnosed with diabetes may feel scared and overwhelmed. Her world has changed, making her suddenly unsure of what she can eat and how to cope with a new illness. In this situation, a Faith Community Nurse could come alongside her and help her learn how to manage her new diagnosis. That may take the form of answering her immediate questions or connecting her with others in the congregation who have already walked that path. It could mean helping her make sense of what this means in her life in terms of her relationship with God.

Or perhaps an older couple is trying to cope with their aging and some of the anxieties that can go with that. Through conversations that encompass both medical and spiritual arenas of concern, Faith Community Nurses can provide support to this couple. Faith Community Nurses have the ideal skill set to provide care coordination that addresses a person's deeper, felt needs because they can take time to listen as they seek to understand what a person's broader concerns are, and help them develop an action plan within the context of their actual resources – physically, emotionally, spiritually, and relationally.

WHY HOSPITALS AND CONGREGATIONS SHOULD CONNECT

Even a cursory review of history indicates that churches have played a major role in supporting people's spiritual and physical health for centuries. During his time on earth, Jesus performed many miracles healing illnesses, and his disciples have followed his example ever since. Before hospitals existed, people turned to churches for care in times of sickness or death.[5] It seems in the past there was a better understanding of the interconnected nature of physical, spiritual, and emotional health than there is in a secular society.

> Hospitals and churches share a common desire to alleviate human suffering. While hospitals today are better equipped to offer acute care, churches still have an important role to play in helping people understand and experience whole-person health.

In fact, if you look at the three major reasons that non-religious people turn to congregations, you will find that all of them include a component of health:

1. **People turn to religion in search of peace.** A woman who has wrestled with a tendency toward depression for her entire life finds herself falling hard and fast after an unexpected divorce. Although there is a clinical element to her condition, she does not realize it yet. Instead of going to a physician, she turns first to the church.

2. **People involve their churches in times of hope and joy.** A couple has had their first child, and in the midst of all the new medical information they have to digest, they are filled with hope and joy at the new birth. One of the ways they may choose to express this is by turning to the church for a baby baptism or dedication.

3. **People turn to faith in times of suffering.** A teenager has been diagnosed with cancer. Chemotherapy is helping his physical condition, but mentally and emotionally, he is struggling to understand why, if God is good, he is allowing this to happen. For answers, he looks to his youth pastor.

Hospitals can address some aspects of these situations and so can congregations, but without a partnership, neither is as effective as they can be together.

WHY THE DISCONNECT?

Hospitals and congregations often remain disconnected because they are not sure how to relate to one another. They do not know what the correct business model or partnership is.

Hospitals have to focus on sustainability, which currently comes from treating patients when they are sick instead of when they are healthy. They are also often afraid that if they try to work with churches, the congregations will perceive it as a type of marketing. Rather than looking for ways to overcome these obstacles, hospitals close the door on any sort of long-term partnership and resort instead to sending out occasional flyers inviting church members to attend a community program.

Hospitals may also struggle to understand from a cultural perspective how to approach and work with different denominations. And, they wonder, even if they did understand, what could they offer that would be helpful? They may feel unsure about what the greatest needs of the congregation are and what a healthy relationship with them would look like. For example, should relationships with congregations fall under the mission and ministries departments or under a clinical or operational area of the hospital?

At the same time, congregations may be afraid to reach out to hospitals because hospitals are often so much bigger than churches. This leaves clergy and congregation members unsure of who to contact and which department they might work in – the chaplain, a marketing person, etc. What can make it even more confusing is that a hospital may have several departments that appear similar to the public. For example, these might have names such as community outreach, community impact, corporate relations, community relations, or community benefit. A person outside of the system might feel overwhelmed just trying to figure out where to begin. Once they finally reach someone at a hospital, many church representatives face a second problem of not knowing what to ask, except for maybe some free items for their health booth, if they have one.

Thus, a lack of communication and education plays a larger role in the separation between churches and hospitals than any difference in culture. Both organizations need someone who understands both systems and can become an effective bridge between them.

FAITH COMMUNITY NURSES CAN BRIDGE THE GAP

Physicians are very focused on disease and treatment, but there is more to a person's experience of illness than the disease itself. To some extent, social workers deal with these other factors – the cost of disease, the types of support available, and various other stressors related to the disease. However, there are limits to what they ordinarily try to help patients and their families deal with. When it comes to emotional needs, for example, patients often turn to therapists, who help them recover a sense of equilibrium, assuming that someone else is taking care of the disease process. The lenses that different medical care providers use to view their patients are often influenced by their specialties.

The situation is different for nurses. In nearly every baccalaureate nursing program, students are required to conduct home visits. As they do, they see the range of how people live. They realize that when a person is sent home from the hospital, they cannot assume there is a bed there. There may not be food in the refrigerator. The children may not have clothing. They cannot assume that just because the surgery was a success that everything is going to go well, because people live in all kinds of situations.

Nurses are also exposed to a wide variety of topics during their training. They study psychology and the human lifespan from birth through death. They learn about home care and acute care. Regardless of what they choose to specialize in after graduating, they know a little bit about a lot of things. They are able to put everything in the context of how people really live.

Since this type of training is similar to that received by most pastors who attend seminary, the nurse and pastor are natural allies in their interest in the needs of the whole person. Although some pastors have not considered health as a theological or spiritual issue, either for themselves or their parishioners, a Faith Community Nurse can connect a pastor with resources that can broaden his or her focus and thus strengthen the ministry that the nurse and pastor share.

Depending on where they work in the public sector, nurses may or may not feel comfortable discussing spiritual things. If they see a rosary at a patient's bedside, for example, some might take it as a clue that there are matters of faith the patient may want to discuss. Others might not know the significance of the prayer beads. When nurses have the opportunity to serve within a congregation, however, they enter a realm of belief and structure that they understand. If congregation, members pray extemporaneously, they are comfortable with that. If in their congregation's culture prayer means reading from a book, they are comfortable with that.

> Faith Community Nurses know what matters to people in their congregations and know how to reach their hearts without having to ask as many questions as an outsider might in order to put the pieces together. Because of this, they can minister naturally to people as their needs require.

PART 2

HOSPITAL AND CHURCH:
CONNECTING TWO DISTINCTIVE WORLDS

The most important thing about Faith Community Nurses is whether or not they are mission-minded individuals who feel a spiritual calling to serve in this capacity.

A BRIEF HISTORY OF FAITH COMMUNITY NURSING

In the 1980s, Chaplain Granger E. Westberg received a grant to establish connections between local congregations and the Lutheran General Hospital in Chicago where he worked. He began by identifying nurses who were interested in trying something new and arranging for them to serve as health ministers in their churches. He gave them the name "Parish Nurses," because local congregations in his denomination (as well as in many other denominations) were called "parishes." Each month this experimental group would meet to provide an update on their successes and struggles. One of the comments that came up frequently was, "I need to know more about how to pray with people and offer them spiritual care."

Westberg realized that while the nurses could easily answer questions about medications and communicate with other care providers, they often felt unsure about how to navigate the spiritual realm. Using the information he gathered from these meetings, Westberg developed a curriculum to equip and train "Parish Nurses," which are referred to in this report as "Faith Community Nurses."

Through the years Westberg's curriculum was refined, and by 1986, Faith Community Nursing became a sustainable model supported by the International Parish Nurse Resource Center. The Health Ministries Association then took it to the next level by organizing an official set of scope and standards of practice for Faith Community Nursing. In 1996, they presented this to the American Nurses Association, the largest professional organization for nurses, who accepted and endorsed it as an official nursing specialty. Because of this, today Faith Community Nursing is recognized with as great a degree of respect as other nursing specialties such as pediatrics, critical care, and geriatric nursing.

Faith Community Nurses combine professional nursing with health ministry. Faith Community Nursing emphasizes health and healing within a faith community. The Faith Community Nurse understands health to be a dynamic process that includes the spiritual, psychological, physical, and social dimensions of the person.

The spiritual dimension is the central core of Faith Community Nurse Practice. Nurses search deep within their souls to find meaning, purpose, and fulfillment in life. By living out their beliefs and faith with self, others, and God, Faith Community Nurses are enabled to offer hope to those they serve. Crisis, illness, and hospitalization can affect one's spiritual wellbeing and quality of life, but as Faith Community Nurses serve with compassion, mercy, and dignity, they exemplify God's love, which can facilitate healing even in the absence of a cure. The Faith Community Nurse serves as:

- Integrator of faith and health

- Provider of spiritual care

- Liaison to community resources and referral agent

- Health counselor, advocate, and educator

- Facilitator of support groups

- Provider of assessment oversight

- Volunteer trainer [6]

FUNDAMENTALS OF FAITH COMMUNITY NURSING

In order to become prepared as a Faith Community Nurse, an individual must hold a current registered nurse license and go through additional education and training. The curriculum is owned by International Parish Nurse Resource Center and approved by the American Nursing Association. Florida Hospital uses this official curriculum and adds additional elements to it. The curriculum used in Florida Hospital's Faith Community Nursing Training includes the following topics:[7]

- **Healing and Wholeness** – The difference between being physically made well and experiencing a sense of wholeness, health, and wellbeing even when an illness is not cured.

- **Applications across Faith Communities** – Understanding the particular beliefs, customs, rituals, and prayers that different faith traditions hold in relation to health, healing, and illness.

- **Health and Wellness in the Faith Community** – The authority for medical ministry in congregations today and the role of the faith community and the Faith Community Nurse to promote health, healing, and wellness.

- **Presence** – Basic concepts of spiritual ministry and guidelines for offering spiritual care.

- **History and Philosophy** – Context on how the nursing profession and different beliefs in God developed.

- **History of Faith Community Nursing** – An overview of the formation and expansion of congregational health ministries in the United States.

- **Philosophy of Faith Community Nursing** – A review of the philosophy of Faith Community Nursing with emphasis on the multiple aspects of the nurse's role in supporting the integration of health ministry into the life of the community of faith.

- **Assessment** – How to use skills of observation, palpation, and auscultation to assess the wholistic health of individuals, families, groups, and the congregation.

- **Self-Care** – The importance of a nurse's caring for himself/herself in order to be fully present and prepared to care for others. Concepts of rest, symptoms of adrenaline high, and ways to become mindful of stressors are explored.

- **Domestic Violence** – The role Faith Community Nurses play in assessing, screening, intervening, and reporting abuse. Spiritual interventions are emphasized.

- **Health Promotion** – How to empower people to take control of and improve their own health.

- **Prayer** – The role prayer plays in the integration of spirituality and health, and ways to use it in ministry.

- **Health Counseling** – How to communicate in a manner that is compassionate, direct, instructive, and ultimately helpful to the one who is receiving counsel.

- **Forgiveness** – How to reframe anger from the past in order to achieve peace in the present and a revitalized sense of purpose for the future.

- **Care Coordination: Volunteers** – How to work with volunteers and support groups.

- **Communication and Collaboration** – How to keep others informed, and how to work well with those who share the mission.

- **Ethics** – How to apply ethical analysis and ethical decision making in various situations.

- **Advocacy** – How to advocate for individuals and families, as well as mobilize the faith community to address health-related issues in need of change.

- **Legal Aspects** – The professional accountability and responsibility of registered nurses as outlined by their specific state nurse practice act and its application to Faith Community Nursing Practice.

- **Referral Agent** – How to make referrals, evaluate various types of referrals based on the size and demographic of the faith community, and how to determine the availability of healthcare resources within the community.

- **Understanding Suffering, Grief, and Loss** – The role religion plays in helping people process and find meaning in death and dying.

- **Documenting Practice** – The importance of documentation and several documentation systems that can be used in Faith Community Nursing practice.

- **Beginning Your Ministry** – Realistic expectations and priorities when first beginning a Faith Community Nurse ministry. Emphasis is placed on the fact that God's timing is often much different than ours; therefore, to have discernment, patience, persistence, and trust is of dire importance.

CASE STUDY – FROM BURNOUT TO BALANCE

The importance of this education and ongoing support for Faith Community Nurses can be seen in the experience of a Faith Community Nurse we'll call "Jenny." Jenny had served as a registered nurse for a number of years before becoming a Faith Community Nurse in a local church. The church in question had a large senior population, and soon after she got started, a number of these seniors passed away. Suddenly a wide variety of people turned to Jenny for emotional, spiritual, and physical support.

"Why is this happening?" they wanted to know. "What am I going to do now? How am I supposed to prepare for a funeral? How am I going to cope with this loss?"

After weeks of sitting at the bedsides of dying church members, providing advice to their family and friends on how to handle medical issues, and comforting people coping with loss, Jenny was burned out.

"I can't do this," she said. "I can't."

Recognizing that she needed help, Jenny called Florida Hospital and asked to be connected with someone who could provide grief support *for her*. The director of pastoral care was happy to help, and after several sessions Jenny was better equipped to provide the same type of support in her church.

Three years later, Jenny is still serving as a Faith Community Nurse and loves her role. In fact, the church has seen so much value in the service she provides that Jenny is now on their staff as an associate minister. It took a strong connection between a hospital and a church to facilitate this type of whole-person healing, a connection that included Faith Community Nurse support meetings and the availability of a variety of wholistic resources and tools.

WHAT FAITH COMMUNITY NURSES DO: PERCEPTION VS. REALITY

Faith Community Nurses are not just people who stop by once in a while to check a church member's blood pressure. They are active participants, present in the daily lives and struggles of fellow congregants. In addition to performing regular nursing activities such as conducting assessments, explaining diagnoses, and guiding members toward solutions, Faith Community Nurses offer spiritual support. With these various roles, confusion can sometimes exist around Faith Community Nursing. Here are some of the most common disconnects between perception and reality.

Perception	Reality
A Faith Community Nurse can replace my medical doctor	A Faith Community Nurse will serve as an advocate for your health and wellness, but cannot provide invasive medical care
Anyone who is a nurse and volunteers in the church is a Faith Community Nurse	Faith Community Nursing is an official recognized sub-specialty of the American Nursing Association that is given at the completion of the Fundamentals of Faith Community Nursing Course
All Faith Community Nurses are employees of a hospital	There are many models of Faith Community Nursing, including volunteer, grant-subsidized, employed by the church, or connected to the hospital
Faith Community Nursing is a program to care for seniors	Faith Community Nurses can provide care for anyone in the congregation, young and old
Faith Community Nurses are here only to take care of my physical health	Faith Community Nurses support the health of body, mind, and spirit
Faith Community Nurses can replace the visiting nurse or hospice	Faith Community Nurses work with agencies in the community for appropriate referrals

FAITH COMMUNITY NURSING MODELS

Faith Community Nursing models vary depending on a church's financial resources and available talent, but in general there are four options.

Option 1 – Congregation Funded

The first is to have a Faith Community Nurse who is paid by the congregation. In this model, the nurse is considered part of the church's staff, and the clergy supervises the spiritual care that he or she provides. When it comes to performing nursing functions, however, the nurse is held accountable according to his or her nursing license.

Option 2 – Volunteer Model

Another option that is frequently used is to have a Faith Community Nurse who is a volunteer from the congregation. In this case the Faith Community Nurse may not have as much time to devote to the role, but all the standards and responsibilities are the same. This model allows nurses who may have other jobs to be able to live out their faith by volunteering as a Faith Community Nurse.

Option 3 – Hospital Sponsored

The third model is the one Faith Community Nursing was originally based on: having a Faith Community Nurse who is paid by the hospital. In the medical world, the first thirty days after someone is discharged from the hospital are a critical period. If the patient is covered by Medicare or Medicaid and is readmitted during that time, the hospital will not be paid for the services it has provided. More importantly, though, it means the patient's health has continued to suffer. Hospitals benefit from employing Faith Community Nurses who can follow up with patients to ensure they understand their discharge instructions and are continuing to improve. The con of this model is that as with all positions in a hospital, the focus can easily shift to accountabilities and return on investment, strategically altering the Faith Community Nurse's role so that it aligns with the hospital's agenda.

Option 4 – Grant Supported

Another model of Faith Community Nursing is one where financial support comes from a combination of grants and the congregation. This model is often employed to help start a new Faith Community Nursing program. In these instances, it is important for congregations to ensure that there is clear leadership ownership and a plan for sustainability in place so that the program does not end when the grant is up.

It is worth noting that some churches also choose to employ Faith Community Nurses who are not from their congregations or even their denomination. For example, one of the original churches that embraced Faith Community Nursing was Lutheran, yet they employed a Roman Catholic Faith Community Nurse, and it worked very well. Some Faith Community Nurses prefer this structure as it makes it easier for them to set boundaries around their time and to enjoy their own time of worship without distraction from well-meaning folks seeking healthcare advice during services.

> The most important thing to consider is not what denomination Faith Community Nurses come from, but whether or not they are mission-minded individuals who feel a spiritual calling to serve in this capacity.

EXPAND YOUR DEFINITION OF "HEALTH"

Too often people limit their view of health to the topics of nutrition and exercise when, in reality, good health encompasses so much more. Florida Hospital describes whole-person health in terms of CREATION Health. This is an acronym for Choice, Rest, Environment, Activity, Trust in God, Interpersonal relationships, Outlook, and Nutrition – all factors that affect our health. Each principle is found in the Creation story as described in the Old Testament book of Genesis.

The chances are if you look at the activities of your church from this perspective, you'll discover that you have already been carrying out a health ministry, whether or not you were aware of it. Do you offer marriage counseling? That helps people improve their Interpersonal relationships and, as a result, their health. Does your church host retreats? That helps people take time to Rest and renew their energy. Do you offer support groups for recovering addicts? That helps people improve their Outlook. Do you hold special prayer meetings or Bible studies? That helps people Trust in God. So, even though these kinds of common church activities or programs may not be classified as health oriented, they really are from a whole-person perspective.

Faith Community Nurses can be helpful in this type of analysis. As part of their fundamental role of conducting assessments, Faith Community Nurses can evaluate individuals, families, or broader groups within your congregation to "diagnose" what the greatest health risks and needs are. They then can "prescribe" a solution that addresses the key issues.

For example, a Faith Community Nurse might conduct a health assessment of your church's youth group and discover that the largest self-identified struggle among those teens is depression. The young people may feel burdened by pressures to get into the "right" college and to fit in to various peer groups. They may see a conflict in the values of their home and church with what they see in their environment. They know they have large decisions to make that will affect their future, and may feel lost. After the assessment, the Faith Community Nurse can create individualized plans to help address the needs and interests of the congregation. This is just one of the ways Faith Community Nurses can add depth and meaning to your church's health ministry while expanding its impact.

Another good starting point for developing a health ministry is to look at your church's mission and vision statement and ask, "What did we say we are here to do?" You will likely find that your organization already has a stated commitment to healing hearts and souls, relieving suffering, or helping people live life to the fullest. Here are some sample mission and vision statements from a variety of religious perspectives:

- To build a healthy community of believers who love each other and love the Torah and mitzvoth (instructions & commands) of our great and awesome God.

- To build a family of devoted followers of Christ that worships God, shares Christ's hope and love, and ministers to each other's needs.

- To serve God through word and witness; to treat all human beings as sisters and brothers; and to foster responsible stewardship of all God's creation.

After examining your organization's mission and vision statement, do a quick assessment of how well your organization is doing at carrying out that mission. Write down any thoughts you have on ways to improve.

Going through these processes has several benefits. First of all, it can help you and others in your congregation better understand the connection between health ministry and the church's stated purpose. It can also help you identify what you are already doing in this arena. This, conversely, will show you where you can improve.

COMMON CONCERNS RELATED TO A
FAITH COMMUNITY NURSE PROGRAM

One of the most common fears churches express when it comes to starting a health ministry or employing a Faith Community Nurse is the fear of lawsuits. It is unfortunate that we live in a day and age when even the best intentions can land people in court. However, the types of things Faith Community Nurses do are not ordinarily subject to malpractice lawsuits. They do not administer medication or perform any types of invasive procedures. As further protection, Faith Community Nurses are urged (sometimes required by their organizations) to carry their own malpractice insurance.

Some churches are also concerned about privacy. Members and even pastors can have a difficult time learning to trust someone new with sensitive information. Fortunately, the topic of privacy is thoroughly covered in the Faith Community Nursing Course. Faith Community Nurses are trained to know what is appropriate and inappropriate to share during prayer requests, or how to respond when stopped in the hall by a church member inquiring about the details of "Mrs. Smith's" health. For example, the rules of the Health Insurance Portability and Accountability Act (HIPAA) require professional confidentiality in relation to such details, so a Faith Community Nurse might say, "I'm not at liberty to discuss the details of Mrs. Smith's health with you, but I'm sure that she would be encouraged to know that you are thinking of her."

One other concern sometimes hinders pastors from supporting the development of a health ministry in their church. This is the concern that launching a health ministry will put another area of their lives under their congregation's scrutiny. Pastors are at the front and center of the church. Too often they are not allowed to make mistakes, and they are not allowed to take a break. They have to be perfect models of spiritual health. If you suggest adding a physical health component to that, some pastors will feel uncomfortable. It is not usually an area they are trained in, and sometimes it is not an area of their personal life they are proud of.

In recent years, the health of pastors has been the subject of increased media coverage and several scientific studies. One article in *The Christian Century* begins, "Being a pastor is bad for your health. Pastors have little time for exercise. They often eat meals in the car or at potluck dinners not known for their fresh green salads. The demands on their time are unpredictable and never ending, and their days involve an enormous amount of emotional investment and energy. Family time is intruded upon. When a pastor announces a vacation, the congregation frowns. Pastors tend to move too frequently to maintain relationships with doctors who might hold them accountable for their health. The profession discourages them from making close friends."[8]

National Public Radio reports, "Priests, ministers, rabbis and imams are generally driven by a sense of duty to answer calls for help. But research shows that in many cases, they rarely find time for themselves. Members of the clergy suffer from [a variety of chronic diseases] and many are burning out."[9]

Here are some facts about the health of pastors:

- In a 2010 survey, the Texas District of the Lutheran Church – Missouri Synod reported, "Over one quarter of [their pastors] (27 percent) report high levels of 'fatigue and irritation' as part of their daily ministry experiences and 26 percent have 'often' or 'very often' felt 'worn out' in the last 30 days."[10]

- An earlier survey of over 17,000 active North Carolina United Methodist clergy showed their rates of obesity to be about 10 percent higher than other North Carolinians, and that clergy rates of high blood pressure and asthma were about 4 percent higher and diabetes rates at about three percent higher than those of their non-clergy peers. In addition, depression rates in pastors, which approach about 10 percent, were roughly double that of all people in the United States.[11]

No one is perfectly healthy, so even pastors can have diabetes, be overweight, or suffer from depression or cardiovascular issues. They may fear being asked health-related questions to which they do not know the answer. All of this can contribute to their reluctance to start a health ministry.

Having a Faith Community Nurse can allay some of that fear because it provides a knowledgeable person to whom members can turn, or be referred, for expert answers in matters of health. Faith Community Nurses exist to support pastors as well, and can provide resources and encouragement to help them boost their own health.

PART 3

Lessons Learned:
Unpacking the Pilot Project

"Having a Faith Community Nurse as part of our congregation makes us all think about health in a different way. It has become part of everything we do, from what we serve at potlucks to what activities we plan for church events."

– Pastor of a Health Ministry Congregation

THE DIFFERENCE ONE FOUNDATION MADE

The Winter Park Health Foundation of Central Florida is a community-based organization whose function is to support the health of the communities they serve. Among three focus areas, one committee is concerned primarily with the health and care of the elderly, and another with the health of the community at large. Both committees decided to experiment with combining their grants for a given time to see if they could fund a bigger project by sharing their resources.

One of the proposed initiatives was for Faith Community Nursing. Because of Florida Hospital's history in this arena, the Winter Park Health Foundation asked the hospital health ministry team to administer the grant. Around the same time, Florida Hospital was developing an initiative called Healthy 100 Churches with a similar purpose. Since these two projects were such a good match, Florida Hospital accepted the opportunity.

As a professor of nursing at the University of Central Florida, Dr. Susan Chase has long held an interest in Faith Community Nursing. When she learned about the project, she saw it as a great opportunity to study a group of congregations that others could learn from. Chase wrote a research proposal for the project and had it approved by the Institutional Review Board of her university, a group that ensures study participants and research data are treated in an ethical manner consistent with the standards set forth in the Helsinki Accords, among others.

Plans were made to establish Faith Community Nursing practices in five churches with the goal of enhancing members' health. All of this was to be done through the connection between faith and healthful living, and connecting hospital and church culture to promote change in each faith community, enabling it to promote healthy living.

From the beginning it was important that each congregation define what success would look like to them. Most assumed that the areas where they would see the biggest differences would be nutrition and physical activity. However, after they conducted a health interest survey, it was clear that the topics their members wanted to learn more about were quite different than what had been expected.

Members were interested in a broad range of subjects, including meditation, laughter, stress management, weight loss, and healthy eating, as well as home and hospital visits, organizing classes, and individual health teaching. Each church used this health interest survey as a basis for addressing their members' individualized needs.

Because we were able to do a third-party study, we can report on activities and now demonstrate the effectiveness or essence of Faith Community Nursing. Before going into those results, though, let's explore a little more about what was done with the grant on the hospital side.

Healthy 100 Church Ministry, the initiative Florida Hospital was in the process of developing before this project began, had three phases. The first phase focused on getting the pastor on board, educated, and inspired about health ministry. The second phase concentrated on information dissemination through training, including studying the official Fundamentals of Faith Community Nursing course. Monthly meetings were held, and a speakers' bureau was developed, along with a variety of online tools and resources that nurses could use. Once the pastor was inspired and on board, and each church had a Faith Community Nurse who was trained, the third phase began. The focus of this phase was to determine how to implement the model in each particular congregation, how the hospital might help in that process, and how to measure and share results.

VARIOUS PERSPECTIVES ON THE DIFFERENCE MADE BY THIS PROJECT

More than once during this project, pastors reported, "Having a Faith Community Nurse as part of our congregation makes us all think about health in a different way. It has become part of everything we do, from what we serve at potlucks to what activities we plan for church events."

Another sentiment that was frequently expressed was, "It makes us comfortable just to know that there is someone we can reach out to if a crisis were to happen or if we have questions." Members from that congregation echoed the pastor's thoughts, saying, "It's good to know there is someone I can ask a question if I really need to, instead of having to wait for a regular doctor's appointment, which may still be two months away."

Across the board congregations expressed feeling a greater sense of support in making health changes and dealing with difficult situations when they had a Faith Community Nurse.

THE VIEW FROM THE MEDIA

Local media – including radio, TV, magazines, and newspapers – are usually interested in stories with a positive message. News about anyone trying to address our world's health crisis is likely to gain an editor's attention, even if the story includes a focus on spiritual as well as physical components of health, since health is a topic on everyone's mind these days.

There are many ways to gain local media attention, any of which can be used to inform the community of your group's interest in helping people improve their health. One Faith Community Nurse wrote a letter to the editor describing her church's creative connection of walking with significant dates on the annual church calendar.

The same newspaper featured an article on the Faith Community Nurse model, with this title: "Growing number of churches hiring nurses to motivate the faithful." Author Kate Santich wrote, "Though religion's role in medicine can be traced to ancient civilizations, churches in more modern times have not always been exemplars of healthy living. [Recently], researchers at Northwestern University reported that young adults who regularly attend religious activities are 50 percent more likely to become obese by middle age than their nonreligious peers. You can blame some of that on church traditions of Sunday morning donuts and fat-laden potluck suppers, particularly in Southern congregations. That's why one mission of faith-community nurses is to encourage more-healthful choices, both at those church get-togethers and at home."[12]

This article was picked up and expanded by the Internet publication, ChurchLeaders.com, quoting one of the nurses in the pilot project, "Parish nursing is different in that it's really promoting wellness, instead of treating someone after they become ill." The nurse described how she urges anyone who will listen on the importance of taking care of themselves. No one is too old or too young to take this message to heart, which is why this nurse once addressed a group of three- and four-year-olds on the topic that "our bodies are a wonderful creation of God."[13]

It's safe to say that when you're trying to make a positive impact in an area like health improvement, you never know who is going to take an interest. In 2010, First Lady Michelle Obama launched a national initiative called *Let's Move*, aimed at reversing the epidemic of childhood obesity. As part of the program, churches across the United States were challenged to become beacons of wellness – getting active, eating healthy, and helping their communities – then to share their stories in the form of a video that would be sent to the First Lady.

One of the churches in the pilot project made a video that showcased their weekly faith and fitness exercise class, the community gardens that they had established, and many other ministry activities that had improved the health of their congregation and community. They were selected as the first-prize winner, and the church's health ministry chairman and Faith Community Nurse were invited to the White House, where they were honored for their efforts to promote wellness in their community.

"With lots of creativity and a great sense of fun, these congregations and organizations have shown us the inspiring work being done across the country to help our children lead healthier lives," said First Lady Michelle Obama. "Everyone wants to see our nation become healthier, and these contest winners have shown us that by taking steps big or small, each of us can play a role in solving the problem of childhood obesity. I hope more people are inspired by these organizations to work together for our children's health."[14]

It is likely that one of the reasons this church won was how they demonstrated a true model of Faith Community Nursing, which is built on connections with a hospital, community resources and agencies, and nonprofits.

THE PASTOR'S VIEW – A CRUCIAL ELEMENT

In any business it is important for the CEO to be on board with a major initiative before it is about to take place. The church pastor, who serves as a kind of CEO for the church, is no different. In order to establish a successful health ministry, pastors have to be enlisted, engaged, educated, and inspired. It helps if they can experience firsthand what a whole-person ministry looks like.

Healthy 100 Churches recently conducted a one-year pilot study called "Rejuvenate," where twenty-five pastors representing six denominations engaged in examining and trying to improve their mental, physical, emotional, and spiritual health. At the beginning, each pastor completed the Celebration Health Assessment at Florida Hospital Celebration Health. This program involves a comprehensive set of tests and screenings that provides a complete update on a person's health status in just one day.[15]

For these pastors, the results were astonishing. One was diagnosed with cancer. Several discovered serious health issues of which they were previously unaware, and all of them had significantly higher stress levels and worse health than many of the CEOs who had completed the same battery of tests. Many factors may have contributed to this, but one of them is that pastors are often so focused on caring for others that they neglect to care for themselves.

> The goal was to help pastors see that they are in high-stress jobs with huge demands, often serving on-call 24/7, so it is essential for them to maintain their health for their own sakes and so they can offer their best to others.

The Florida Hospital health ministry team gave them more than facts; they were given resources and experiences aimed at making a difference.

From an organizational standpoint, each element of CREATION Health was considered, with a view toward how help could be provided to that area of pastors' lives. For example, how could the hospital help improve pastors' Outlook or Interpersonal relationships? For this, free, unlimited counseling sessions were provided through a third-party organization called Care for Pastors. Many of the pastors used this for marriage counseling, although they were free to discuss any topic they wanted.

And what about Rest? For the average church attendee, Saturday or Sunday is a meant to be a day of rest, but it is the day when pastors work the hardest, so when do they get a day of rest? Through dialogue with the participants, it was learned that most of them had not taken a day off, yet alone a weekend or week off, for a very long time – some for years. To remedy this, a vacation was made available for them to take with their spouses. The pastors later said the experience was a huge eye-opener to them about their own health and work-life balance. One pastor who had been married for thirty years said he had not spent that much time with his wife since their honeymoon.

By the end of the year-long *Rejuvenate* experience, every participating pastor better understood the connection between mind, body, and spirit, and they were all supportive of the concept of health ministry. In fact, several of them went on to work with their Faith Community Nurses on achieving additional personal goals such as reducing their stress levels or losing weight.

A SAMPLING OF PROGRAMS AND SERVICES

With the five churches participating in the pilot project, there was a wide variation of activities and participation based on the culture of each congregation. In one, health-related programs took precedence. In another, individual spiritual care became the main feature. Some programs were in place before funding was available, and others were started using grant funds. Some Faith Community Nurses and some clergy had experience with health-related programs in other places, while some were entirely new to this arena. As the following examples show, Faith Community Nursing will look different in every congregation, and there is not a right or wrong way to carry out the ministry. Every congregation provides a range of programs and services that are responsive to its own internal and external environment. The next section describes the range of programs and services that were seen in the churches.

HEALTH ACTIVITIES FOCUS

Walking Program: "Walking to Bethlehem" is a program that one church conducted during the season of Advent, a time some congregations spend preparing to celebrate the nativity of Jesus at Christmas. Whenever congregation members went walking, they would record either their pedometer steps or the number of minutes they walked and turn it in to the Faith Community Nurse, who tracked their progress on a map in the church lobby. Their goal was to "walk" from their city to Bethlehem by crossing the ocean, landing in Morocco, and covering the rest of the distance to their destination. The congregation was very engaged with this initiative, and it got them to do something that was healthy during one of the seasons that can be unhealthy with all the parties and good food that the holidays can bring. Because they had such success, other churches have also started using this program, in some cases modifying the theme. For example, one church turned it into a "Walk to Jerusalem" program around Easter.

Exercise Class: Recognizing that they were located in a lower income community where the diabetes rate is twice the national average, one church's leaders decided to focus on weight loss initiatives. They began advertising a weekly faith and fitness exercise class to the public, and achieved a large number of attendees each week. Many of these attendees reported that the social support from the church made the energy of the class feel positive and guilt-free as opposed to a finger-shaking environment where they were told they needed to get moving and lose weight. For example, if a participant arrived a few minutes early, they might hear people say, "Let's go have some fun!"

Community Walk: One church's pastor started a weekly walk with the mayor. The entire congregation was invited to participate in this activity, which provided an opportunity to move and ask questions of key church and civic leadership. Since then health and fitness have become such an integral part of everything this church does that it is not uncommon to hear members refer to their bodies as temples of God.

COMMUNITY EVENTS FOCUS

Providing Food Assistance: One church that was neither large nor wealthy had a desire to help and serve their community. Every Sunday morning they offered a free pancake breakfast to homeless men, making sure these individuals felt welcome to join in the worship services afterward. During the week, the Faith Community Nurse also oversaw a large food pantry to assist those who were struggling.

Offering Free Classes: Another successful activity organized by a church was a laughter-yoga class, which was advertised to the broader community. So many people showed up for the class that the church began offering it twice a day: once for those who were available early on and another for those who couldn't make it until the evenings. While in some cases outreach is used as a growth device, for this church it was truly about being a ministry and a resource to the community.

Raising Awareness: One nurse did a lot in terms of social justice. For example, she sponsored a program to address human trafficking, which is a big issue in Florida, by coordinating with law enforcement personnel, social services, and different healthcare providers. As a result, the church developed an increased sensitivity for counselors and law enforcement officials, and became more aware of what to look for and what resources to engage should human trafficking be suspected. By convening the day-long conference, the church was supporting the health of the community.

PERSONAL MEDICAL CONCERNS FOCUS

Home Visits: One church that was new to the idea of Faith Community Nursing benefitted greatly just from having a medical professional in their congregation to whom they knew they could turn for help. Ever since someone had died during a church service, there existed among the members a certain tentativeness and fear about what would happen in an extreme medical situation.

Because of this, the Faith Community Nurse focused a lot on addressing physical health concerns and visiting people in their homes. Members reported that she actually "saved lives," and they felt very strongly about the positive impact she was able to help them achieve with their health. The pastor said, "Knowing there was a capable nurse who could face any challenge did a lot to make the congregation feel comforted and supported."

A PRIMARILY SPIRITUAL FOCUS

One of the nurses in the pilot stepped into a well-established Faith Community Nursing program. Because the ministry was already underway, she quickly found that members really appreciated having visits from the Faith Community Nurse from whom they received spiritual care and support. A large part of her role became checking on members in the hospital or accompanying people to therapy appointments, but she also offered a deeply pastoral ministry through her presence and encouragement.

An Unexpected Result – The Nurse as a Stabilizing Factor

Several of the churches participating in the pilot experienced significant staff turnover, one having multiple changes in pastoral leadership in the course of three years. During this time, the Faith Community Nurse became the glue of the church. Members felt comfortable talking with her when it seemed no one else was there.

In spite of the challenges inherent in multiple staff changes in any church, the Faith Community Nurse ministry flourished beautifully – proof that even if you anticipate staff changes, it's not necessary to postpone starting a health ministry. If anything, a Faith Community Nurse can serve as a stabilizing force during times of change.

SPECIFIC DATA FROM FAITH COMMUNITY NURSE REPORTS

As part of the pilot project, Faith Community Nurses reported their activities to the Project Coordinator. Activities performed by Faith Community Nurses in five congregations in three, six-month periods are summarized in Table 1.

Nurses engaged in listening and support activities with individual congregation members, taught classes, offered spiritual support, and provided educational materials in church, home, and hospital settings. They engaged with other service providers in the community and provided a connection to other resources available to members, touching hundreds of lives.

Looking at the activities of the Faith Community Nurses from the perspectives of the varied congregations gives a different view. In surveys completed by members in each of the five congregations, members reported what activities of the Faith Community Nurse they had experienced. Table 2 lists major reported activities from the perspective of the congregation members. The survey asked if they had participated once, more than once, or not at all. For "more than once" the number counted was two. The total number of times an activity was counted is reflected in the table.

One major group of activities congregation members reported experiencing was visits. During these visits, a variety of interventions were delivered, including support in learning to manage health conditions, active listening, and spiritual care.

Table 1
Faith Community Nurse Reported Activity Trends
Time Frame: Initial 18-Month Period

Activities/Visits	Months 1 – 6	Months 7 – 12	Months 13 – 18	Totals
Home Visit	40	115	88	243
Hospital Visit	47	90	44	181
Nursing Home Visit	36	63	29	128
Office Visit	113	182	107	402
Telephone Visit	107	118	94	319
Referrals				
Agency	27	31	28	86
Clergy	7	7	10	24
ER	3	4	2	9
MD	27	25	31	83
Other	39	48	19	106
Interventions				
Active Listening	269	415	267	951
Bibliotherapy/ Health Material	85	133	105	323
Counseling	83	64	71	218
Emotional Support	217	371	239	827
Individual Teaching	66	93	103	262
Learning Facilitation	74	86	94	254
Presence	191	323	214	728
Spiritual Support	173	276	178	627
Support System Enhancement	182	304	167	653

Table 2
FCN Activities Reported by Congregation Members

Reported Experience	Total
Activities/Visits	
Blood pressure check	106
Home visit	36
Hospital visit for me	29
Hospital visit for family	29
Health-related class	123
Referrals	
Arrange healthcare appointments	42
Attending a health professional office visit	34
Health Management	
Help with understanding how to maintain health	124
Help understanding management of new condition	78
Help understanding management of chronic condition	75
Help planning long-term care decisions	62
Spiritual Care	
Spiritual care visit	55

SUMMARY OF FINDINGS ON
FAITH COMMUNITY NURSING PROJECT

Data sources for this evaluation include interviews with Faith Community Nurses and clergy from all parishes receiving support; questionnaire data from four of the five congregations, which include the Faith Community Nurse activity questionnaire, open-ended questions on the connection between faith and health, and the respondents' statement of the value of the Faith Community Nurse to their health; and survey data from the Medical Outcomes Survey SF-12 and the Spiritual Wellbeing Scale.[16] One congregation had transitions of both Faith Community Nurse and clergy, and the survey cycle was postponed until a new clergy person became established. The Faith Community Nurse role in that church was filled by one of the Faith Community Nurses who was also working with another of the supported congregations.

Congregation members clearly recognized that prayer, health classes, help in understanding how to maintain personal health, and blood pressure checks were central activities of the Faith Community Nurse. Their report of activities is consistent with activities reports of the Faith Community Nurses.

In addition to the checklist, congregation members wrote in answers to a question on their survey, "What would you like to tell about your experience with your Faith Community Nurse?" Selected responses are listed below:

- *A positive, beneficial experience with some helpful suggestions and encouragement to stay physically and mentally active.*
- *Our Faith Community Nurse is a wonderful, spiritually gifted individual. She speaks clearly about medical and health issues. I consider her a real partner in my health journey.*
- *She has been a consistent help to my family and me as I've gone through heart surgery and my mother's long-term suffering and death.*
- *She is <u>available</u>. She answers phone calls and returns messages and is that "very present help in times of trouble, to quote the psalmist."*

A major feature of all the Faith Community Nurse programs was health programming. One clergy participant reported, "Overall, I think that we're more aware of our health and of our need to be healthy." Another said:

We had a case in our congregation of someone who wasn't doing their medications correctly and had become literally overdosed and really wasn't aware of it. I remember the day that I stood out in the parking lot with this parishioner and she didn't remember how she got to the parking lot. To me, it looked like she was having a stroke. It would have been those sorts of indicators. Our Faith Community Nurse happened to be there. I asked her to come out and we talked and spent time with the parishioner.

Other programs included several from the Healthy 100 Churches program list. In fact, one Faith Community Nurse reported that the Healthy 100 Churches program connection was a benefit overall in that, "I think it does help with my credibility here. People feel as though we are part of a larger institution."[17]

In the congregation survey, one respondent said that they pray for health more now than they had in the past. Another reported having blood pressure monitored and receiving advice about a physical problem. One person wrote, "I like that [the Faith Community Nurse] is spreading the word about healthy living to our congregation. There are many struggling with being overweight, and the activities planned have helped show how little changes can have a big impact." This same person reported that her workout became "a time of prayer and meditation." Another person reported that "our Faith Community Nurse is creative and very thoughtful. She responded to our congregation's needs assessment for activities and stress-reduction with Laughter Yoga." Another person was grateful for the informative articles in the church bulletin.

Two different clergy reported a feeling that one benefit is in the confidence in the membership that comes from knowing the Faith Community Nurse is available, even if not everyone needs the support offered at any given time. Another clergyman reported:

What I see is we've got a very strong health cabinet and having a Faith Community Nursing program has allowed some gifts to come out of the woodwork that would not have come out in the congregation too. So I think those side benefits are huge, as well as the direct ministry.

Overall, health effects are evident in the congregations with active Faith Community Nurse programs. In many, the indirect sense of trust in the support that the Faith Community Nurse could provide if needed were also a source of confidence and security.

FAITH AND SPIRITUALITY

Health-related programming is never done only for itself. Faith Community Nurses do all that they do through a perspective of Faith and Health. One clergyman reported an important aspect of Faith Community Nurse service to the congregation as "to receive the love, care, and compassion, which is in my experience, vital to the healing process, as is prayer itself."

One Faith Community Nurse expressed it this way:

People are really appreciative when I go to their home or hospital visit and I don't come in with a bag of what I want to do, what they need. They open up and I just basically listen. And then, the prayer time... All I do is repeat to them what they've said about their concerns. And then, kind of tie that all together in my head as to what I think might be going on – anxiety or worries about the family I might leave behind, that type of thing. And then, another thing that I find to be powerful is when I put the cross on their forehead. It's a meaningful thing ... And I tell them they are a child of God.

One Faith Community Nurse reported regarding the congregation that "their understanding [is that] they are created uniquely, and also that they can take an active part in trying to maintain their health."

Prayer is essential. One clergyman described the growth of the Faith Community Nurse in terms of leading prayer in public places. In her expanding role, this was an important new skill. He described her "going out and being able to have conversations outside the realm of the spiritual, but yet connected with the spiritual. I won't say that this [validates] her health conversations with parishioners, but it's helpful."

The spiritual life of the Faith Community Nurse is central to the work, as one of them expressed:

I don't think my faith has changed, but I do think I depend on it more for a lot of reasons. You know, you see people die. It's hard to see a lot of loss, and so I really depend on that closeness with the Lord to be able to do this work.

A survey respondent stated:

My faith is paramount to my health because my body is God's temple and I have to take care of it. I believe that how I take care of my body is directly correlated with how I feel about my relationship with God.

Overall Health Outcomes

One feature of the evaluation project was looking at health indicators for congregation members. Two research instruments that have been used in multiple settings were part of the Faith Community Nurse Survey. The SF-12® Health Survey presents individual and group reports that compare respondents' answers with nationally normed data, with a consideration of age and gender.[18] Several variables are measured, but reported here in Table 3 are the Physical Component Scale (which include physical functioning, role performance related to physical health, and bodily pain), and the Mental Component Scale (vitality, social functioning, role performance due to emotional health, and mental health and mean age of respondents by site).

All congregations showed a lower risk for depression as compared with population norms. This would indicate that mental health, vitality, and social function are higher than would be expected in the congregation.

Table 3

Medical Outcomes Survey for Physical and Mental Components of Health

Survey	Percentile
SF-12 Physical Component Scale	51
SF-12 Mental Component Scale	55

The sample for this evaluation was a convenience sample and may have excluded the oldest and sickest members of the congregations. The normed scores take age into account. It is evident that for the total sample, physical health is slightly higher than the national average and that mental health is higher than the average. The scores are quite similar across congregations, with one congregation reporting a higher mental component scale as compared with others.

Table 4

Spiritual Wellbeing

Spiritual Wellbeing	Mean score
SWB Religious Wellbeing	56/60
SWB Existential Wellbeing	53/60
SWB Spiritual Wellbeing	109/120

The Religious, Existential, and overall Spiritual Wellbeing scores were developed using the Spiritual Wellbeing Scale©.[19] Scores were equal to or higher than reported scores of comparable groups. The evaluation study design does not allow for any causal statements. However, the snapshot of reported health for congregation members who chose to answer indicates that they are somewhat healthier than national averages in physical, mental, and spiritual health.

PART 4:

DEFINING SUCCESS:
WHAT YOU CAN DO

As you develop a health ministry, you will likely find that you already

have programs in place that support certain elements of whole-

person health. Use these as a starting point for your health ministry,

refocusing or regrouping them as necessary.

HOW TO ESTABLISH A HEALTH MINISTRY THAT WILL OUTLAST YOU

The first three sections of this report have focused on the pilot project and its results. While a great deal may be gleaned from that information, this final section aims to address these questions:

- How can you use what you've learned about networking hospitals and churches within your arena of influence, for the good of your community?

- How can a sustainable health ministry be established so it will continue into the future even if you are no longer personally involved?

In addition, the Appendix contains a number of tools and resources that were used in the pilot project. You are free to use and adapt these for your own purposes.

Three keys to sustainability are time, talent, and treasure. Everyone – including clergy, nurses, and congregation members – has the opportunity to contribute in one or more of these areas. This last category is often the one people are most uncomfortable with. Although they recognize that income is necessary to provide for their own personal needs, they get uneasy with the idea of linking mission and money in a church situation. These two elements are critical, however, to having a thriving health ministry.

When asking for any of these three T's – time, talent, or treasure – make sure to connect the purpose behind money and mission. One way to do this is by using the Head, Heart, Hand Approach.

Head: What are the facts?

Heart: Why does it matter?

Hand: How can the congregation help?

For example, you may discover during your church's health assessment that many of your members are at risk for heart disease. Your health ministry team would like to address this issue, but they lack the funds to do it. Here is how you can use the Head, Heart, Hand Approach to help your congregation understand the connection between mission and money.

Head: One in four Americans die of heart disease.

Heart: Out of our 500 congregation members, that is 125 of us – on average, one person in every immediate family.

Hand: We need to raise funds for more blood pressure cuffs so that we can all become more aware of our blood pressure, one of the major predictors of heart disease.

CONNECT WITH YOUR HOSPITAL

Regardless of the size of your local hospital, they have key resources they can often offer to support your Faith Community Nurse and health ministry. Look for a particular person to connect with, whether it's a chaplain, a case manager, a nurse, or an admission coordinator. These are the individuals who can serve as guides to the various resources and programs – volunteer groups, health visitors, and so forth – that the hospital has to offer.

When you approach them, however, do not just think about what is in it for your church. Consider ways that your congregation could become a benefit to the hospital and their initiatives. Often the biggest need hospitals have is help in communicating to churches about their like-minded, mission-focused events. A good connection with them can go a long way toward enhancing your health ministry efforts, but it is important that the partnership is mutually beneficial and not just a one-sided connection.

TREAT THE PASTOR LIKE A CEO

As leaders of their congregations, pastors are crucial to ensuring a program's success. The three key elements for treating a pastor like a CEO are to provide inspiration, education, and experience. How those play out will look different in every church and community. The important thing is to recognize the types of stresses pastors are under, and as you go through these steps, treat them with exceptional kindness and respect.

Inspiration comes from helping the pastor see how a focus on health is part of a ministry to the whole person, and of great spiritual significance for those who are seeking to love God with their mind, spirit, and body. In addition, a pastor may be energized by the realization that outreach to the community through a focus on health can be a creative way to open up dialogue about what living life "to the fullest" really means.

Education comes from understanding the roots of the church and its long-established tradition of providing physical and spiritual care to people in need. It is also helpful for pastors to realize that Faith Community Nursing is an official specialty of the American Nursing Association and that special training exists to prepare nurses to serve in a church setting.

Experience comes from providing pastors with the opportunity to see how whole-person care can make a difference in their own lives. Receiving care – emotionally, physically, and spiritually – is something they are often unused to because they are so dedicated to caring for others. But when their own health and wellbeing are supported, they will want to see their people receive similar support as well.

LET YOUR LIGHT SHINE!

As you go about establishing a vibrant health ministry led by a Faith Community Nurse, look for opportunities to promote what you are doing, both internally and externally. Whether you have a small, medium, or large church, there are likely multiple venues that you can use to shine a light on what you are doing: bulletins, newsletters, pre-sermon announcements, websites, and so forth.

Keep in mind that people outside of the church are fascinated by the connection between faith and health as well. Local newspapers, television, and radio stations are always looking for interesting content to feature. As you live and breathe health ministry, stories will naturally come out of your experiences. Do not be shy about sharing them! They are good not only for marketing activities taking place within your church, but also for helping people understand your church culture as a whole.

Another strategy is to watch for opportunities to participate in community events such as large community health fairs, hospital community events, and the city or county's department of health initiatives. These are ideal places to reach new people. Conversations about health are not difficult to initiate, even with strangers, since health is on everyone's mind and is more or less a neutral topic.

ENSURE THE FAITH COMMUNITY NURSE IS CONNECTED TO A BROADER GROUP

Faith Community Nurses can feel very isolated if they do not know anyone else who serves in the same role. Being part of regional groups can help them grow and get support for what they are doing from other people who are doing a similar kind of work. They can also share ideas, resources, and success stories. If no local groups are available, encourage them to connect to a larger organization such as the Health Ministries Association or the International Faith Community Nursing Resource Center for more national support.[20]

RECOGNIZE THE CALLING

While there are many business aspects of Faith Community Nursing, at the end of the day it is important to understand that Faith Community Nursing is not a career; it's a calling with a major ministry component. In fact, many individuals who become Faith Community Nurses say, "This is what I came into nursing for in the first place. I want to be with people, and I felt called into this role."

If your church has a special recognition of ministry, such as a "Blessing of the Hands" (a prayer of blessing for those who serve), you might consider including your Faith Community Nurse in it. Use the opportunity to dedicate the person and the effort, much like you might do when commissioning a missionary to some foreign land. The only difference is that the "mission field," in this case, is your parish, congregation, or the community you serve. Affirming your Faith Community Nurse will make it clear to your entire congregation that he or she is an official part of your spiritual care team.

PULL TOGETHER EXISTING PROGRAMS

As you develop a health ministry, examine through a CREATION Health lens the activities you already offer that relate to one's mind, body, spirit, or relationships. You will likely find that you already have programs in place that support certain elements of whole-person health. Use these as a starting point for your health ministry, refocusing or regrouping them as necessary. The following list is a compilation of various programs typically sponsored by churches to build relationships among members based on their common interests or needs. All of these have a potential connection to one or more of the letters that make up the acronym CREATION Health:

____ Healthy Lifestyle Study Groups
____ Creation Care
____ Weight Loss
____ Fitness
____ Marriage Classes
____ Pre-Marriage Classes
____ Divorce Care
____ Grief & Loss
____ New Believers Groups
____ Women's Bible Studies
____ Men's Bible Studies
____ Parenting Groups
____ Anger Management
____ Single Parenting
____ Aging Parent(s) Care
____ Single Adults
____ Prayer Groups
____ Parenting
____ Ministry to the Disabled
____ Breast Cancer Survival
____ Healing Ministry
____ Healthy Cooking
____ English as a Second Language

____ Health Care Clinic for
         the Underserved
____ Financial Classes
____ Jail Ministry
____ Mentoring Teens
____ Homeless Ministry
____ Mission Trips
____ Crisis Management Groups
____ Neighborhood/Community
         Outreach Groups

Special Interest Groups:
____ Art Group
____ Financial Advisors
____ Motorcycle Group
____ Softball Team
____ Tennis
____ Word Weavers
____ Home Educators
____ Disaster Recovery Team
____ Gardening
____ Bird Watching
____ Exploring Creation

Take a moment and, using the list above, place any letter from the CREATION acronym next to each small group or special interest group. Remember that C = Choice; R = Rest; E = Environment; A = Activity; T = Trust in God; I = Interpersonal Relationships; O = Outlook; N = Nutrition. Since it's usually easier to redirect an entity in motion, this overall view of what's already happening in your setting could provide some insight into where you could start.

BUILD A STRONG TEAM

As wonderful as it is to have a Faith Community Nurse, it takes more than one person to have a successful health ministry. Make sure you encourage other people in your congregation to get involved on the team. This is one way to support the sustainability of the health ministry so when one or more health ministry team leaders are absent, the health programs will keep running. Having a team also provides the opportunity for Faith Community Nurses to focus on their calling and their specialty of nursing, while the team takes care of the health promotion and programmatic elements. It is a win for everybody. If you are interested in learning how to start a health ministry team in your church, visit www.Healthy100Churches.com.

DEFINE SUCCESS FROM THE BEGINNING

One of the keys to achieving success is knowing how to recognize it, which is impossible if you do not first talk about what it looks like. From the beginning it is important to sit down with your team and ask, what is the purpose of our health ministry? How does this tie in with the mission statement of our church? What programs are we going to be running? What expectations do we have for the Faith Community Nurse?

All of the churches in the pilot project were successful in different ways. The ones that had the most quantitative data to demonstrate success were the ones who stuck most closely to the plans they developed based on their health interest survey results. For example, if congregation members identified on the survey that stress management was one of their biggest areas of concern and the church focused on that, it was easy for them to measure success. Had the church decided to focus on another area, they might not have had as much participation, and as a result, their numbers would not have reflected as great a change.

It is easy to look around a congregation and say, "They need a weight loss program." But if you survey that congregation and the members respond that weight loss is not a priority for them, the chances of them participating in any weight-loss centric activities you plan is low. Since attending a church program is voluntary, if members do not perceive value, they will not come. Do not waste your time, talent, and treasure trying to guess what people are interested in. Base your direction on the results of the health interest survey, and make sure you define from the beginning how you will know you have reached the goal.

ESTABLISH BOUNDARIES TO PROTECT YOUR FAITH COMMUNITY NURSE

During the process of defining success, take time to also determine what your expectations are for the Faith Community Nurse in terms of time and contributions. Communicating this clearly from the beginning will help your Faith Community Nurse establish healthy boundaries so that they are not working twenty-four hours a day, seven days a week. One way to do this is by establishing and posting Faith Community Nurse "office hours" through bulletins and church newsletters. By maintaining continuous reporting of hours, they can monitor themselves to ensure they are keeping to their limits. That is often the most difficult aspect of Faith Community Nursing.

MOST IMPORTANTLY ... SEEK GOD'S GUIDANCE

Having a health ministry and Faith Community Nurse can make a huge difference in your congregation and community. You don't want to embark on this journey lightly, though. It is always important to ask for God's direction. Like any ministry, you will need spiritual wisdom and guidance on the process, so make sure that this is a matter of prayer among your staff and within your congregation, not just before you begin, but as your health ministry helps your people become healthier.

CONCLUSION:
EXTENDING THE HEALING MINISTRY OF CHRIST

At the end of the day, Faith Community Nursing is not about streamlined processes or hitting financial savings targets. It is about caring and touching the hearts of people who are going through traumatic, sometimes devastating, life experiences. Earlier we introduced you to Jenny, a Faith Community Nurse who found that she needed support herself and wisely reached out for it when a wave of deaths took place at her church. Through grief counseling she regained her energy and was even better prepared to make sense of and deal with loss.

Through regular visits, Jenny became very close to an elderly woman in her congregation whom we will call Carolyn. For months, Jenny witnessed Carolyn suffering from end-stage renal disease. Jenny came to know firsthand the ups and downs of battling with this illness, and the discomfort that can accompany a treatment plan that includes various types of therapy. Jenny could see that Carolyn's energy and vitality were waning, and she knew that Carolyn sometimes wondered "What's the point?" even as friends and family members encouraged her to push on and "beat this thing."

One day during a difficult physical therapy session, Jenny looked at Carolyn and saw the pain etched on her face. She could tell that Carolyn was tired – not the kind of tired easily remedied by a good night's sleep. It was a deep, soul-weariness, the type experienced by one whose days are filled with more pain than joy.

Right there in the chaos of clinicians running around and other patients receiving care, Jenny leaned over and whispered a prayer in Carolyn's ear, and then said, "It's okay," as she put her arm around her. "We don't have to do this." Immediately, she felt Carolyn's muscles relax and a look of peace replace the pain that had been etched on her face just moments before. Carolyn looked at her and nodded.

It was the permission she had needed, the permission that loving family members and friends who wanted to hang on to her as long as possible would never be able to give. Permission that doctors and clinicians, trained and paid to fight to the last, could not offer her. Permission that only one who was closely acquainted with Carolyn's body, spirit, and mind could give. Jenny felt the rightness of the moment, and she knew it was time.

Carolyn spent the next two weeks in hospice with Jenny at her side. This Faith Community Nurse, who a few years before was ready to quit because she did not know how to cope with the deaths of so many members of her congregation, was now able to minister in a beautiful and grace-filled way to a woman in her last days. Instead of carrying her burden of illness with pain and fear, Carolyn departed with a sense of peace and hope, not hope for brighter days here on earth, but for what was to come.

This willingness to walk with someone through the journey of life, and caring for them spiritually, mentally, and physically, is the essence of Faith Community Nursing.

PART 5:

RESOURCES:
TOOLS TO HELP GROW
A HEALTH MINISTRY

The tools and resources included in this Appendix were used in the

pilot program. Feel free to adapt them for your own purposes.

RESOURCE A:

SAMPLE FAITH COMMUNITY NURSE JOB DESCRIPTION

Job Title: Faith Community Nurse/Manager of Health Ministry*

Description: This is a paid position with administrative responsibility for Faith Community Nursing, which is an official specialty recognized by the American Nursing Association.

Reporting Relationship: Executive Pastor, Pastor of Congregational Care, etc.

Purpose: This position holds the responsibility for Faith Community Nursing ministry, which includes: operations and program development of Faith Community Nurse ministry; development of policies and procedures that describe the operations of Faith Community Nursing services; infrastructure within the ministry of the congregation; budget and long-range strategic planning. Additional responsibilities include management of the selection, supervision, continuing education of health ministry team; theological reflection, program development and evaluation of the Faith Community Nursing ministry.

Accountabilities and Job Activities:

I.   Administration

    a.   Administer and document the operations of Faith Community Nursing Ministry, including but not limited to the following:

        i.   Philosophy

        ii.   Mission

        iii.   Vision

        iv.   Theological reflection

        v.   Continuing education

        vi.   Long-range planning

        vii.   Short and long-term goals

        viii.   Organizational chart

        ix.   Practice standards

        x.   Policies and procedures

        xi.   Contracts

        xii.   Evaluation

b. Establishes Health Ministry Team and participates as an advisor and participant member. May chair until administrator of team can be found.

c. Collaborates with pastor/ministry leaders in the development and implementation of a plan to integrate Faith Community Nursing and whole-person care into the continuum of ministries offered.

d. Develops a congregational plan and membership survey tool(s) that evaluates needs, outlines interventions to meet needs, develops membership plan that is inclusive, measures outcomes, modifies ministry and roles.

e. Provides for the evaluation of Faith Community Nursing services and ministry.

II. Inter-program Consultation

a. Collaborates with other leaders within the congregation's ministry to develop relationships that will foster support for whole-person health, Faith Community Nursing services, a healthier congregation, and a healthier community.

b. Represents Faith Community Nursing services at congregation and community service functions.

c. Promotes the development of a health ministry through the development of protocols for working within the congregation.

III. Education and Research

a. Develops and participates in the orientation and education of the pastors, ministry leaders, and membership to Faith Community Nursing and whole-person health within the congregation.

b. Provides for the Faith Community Nurse to attend and participate in annual education and retreats that relate to improving skills within the Faith Community Nursing profession and aspects of spiritual care.

c. Develops and/or participates in research related to Faith Community Nursing and health ministry outcomes.

IV. Program Administration

    a. Develops a long-range strategic plan for the growth and development of Faith Community Nursing services.

    b. Completes an annual evaluation of the Faith Community Nurse ministry in conjunction with the pastor of the congregation.

    c. Directs Faith Community Nursing Services

        i.   Consults with others for new or existing ministries that relate to aspects of whole-person health within the congregation

        ii. Records activities and documents interactions with clients according to Faith Community Nursing guidelines

        iii. Responsible for managing time and fiscal management of the Faith Community Nurse ministry

        iv. Supervises volunteers and health ministry team activities within scope of assignments

    d. Guides congregations in the development of a new health ministry and Faith Community Nurse program

    e. Creates ongoing program status reports to the pastor and leadership administration

V. Grant Administration

    a. Develops grant proposals in collaboration with staff

    b. Maintains accurate records of grant activities in accordance with grant specifications

    c. Develops a documentation system for Faith Community Nursing services

    d. Presents findings developed through grant-funded projects at conferences and through publication

VI. Professional Development

    a. Serves on designated committees within the healthcare system

    b. Represents the healthcare institution at community forums and both internal and external educational programs.

Role Definition:
1. To integrate faith and health in order that the church becomes a place of healing and wholeness;
2. Provides spiritual care intentionally;
3. Assessment of both groups and individuals;
4. Liaison to community resources for appropriate referrals;
5. Referral agent;
6. Provide health counseling;
7. Facilitate health education;
8. Facilitate support groups;
9. Facilitate membership training;
10. Empowerment for congregation to take ownership of life wholistically.

Skill/Education Level:
1. Six or more years of clinical nursing experience
2. Attendance at a Basic Faith Community Nurse Preparation Course using curriculum provided by Florida Hospital;
3. Preferred experience in developing and offering education programs;
4. Excellent communication skills, both oral and written;
5. Experience working with congregations; i.e. has mature faith journey with God and understands faith community in terms of ministry and its ongoing development;
6. Graduate from an accredited school of nursing and maintains a current state RN license.

* Some terminology used in this job description is specific to Florida Hospital. You may adapt or customize to fit your own situation and needs.

RESOURCE B:

WHERE TO LOOK FOR FAITH COMMUNITY NURSING GRANTS

Nearly every major city in the United States has a United Way, Center for Nonprofits, or other centralized organization whose mission is to provide support and resources to nonprofits. Typically, these organizations have a paid subscription to grant databases such as The Foundation Center (www.foundationcenter.org) that community members are allowed to use onsite (just like using resource material at a public library) or they can at least get you started knowing where to look and what is available in the local community. You can also find places to access The Foundation Center grant database by visiting www.grantspace.org and entering your zip code.

If you're looking for a free place to search for grants, try www.grants.gov. This website enables you to enter key words such as "Faith Community Nursing" or "Parish Nursing" and select other criteria that can help narrow down a list of possible matches. A simple web search with the same key words can also pull up a wide variety of resources, although it may take longer to filter through these than if you use a dedicated grant database.

There are three tips to keep in mind when looking for grants. The first is that there are many people and organizations that want to improve their community and are just waiting for a great idea that they can invest in. Some are even under a deadline to give a certain amount of money away each year. If you can dream big for your Faith Community Nurse and health ministry team, someone else has already made up their mind that they want to fund it; you just have to find them.

The second tip that will help you in this process is to read all of the directions on a grant application and stay organized. Each one has a different set of criteria and deadlines. If one seems to match your goals in every way except it says, "Not available for churches," do not waste your time filling out an application. Focus on the grants that are most attainable, and set up a schedule to help you meet all of the deadlines.

Remember as you are filling out your grant application to use the Head, Heart, Hand approach. Think of the people who are reading your application as if they are your church members. They need to be convicted in the same way that you know what you are doing, will be a responsible steward of the resources given to you, and that the project is guaranteed to make a difference in the lives of countless individuals.

RESOURCE C:

SAMPLE SELF-INTEREST SURVEY

Healthy 100 Church Ministry has developed a survey that congregation members can take to give their Faith Community Nurse and ministry leaders a better picture of where they are at and how to serve them in their health journey. The statements below are excerpted from the three sections of this survey.[21]

Section 1: Basic Information

1. Age:
2. Sex:
3. Marital Status:
4. Health Insurance Status:
5. If our church wanted to send out information about activities, news, and tips about healthy living, what would be your preferred way to get that information? (Select all that apply)
   a. Pastor Announcement
   b. Bulletin Board
   c. Weekly E-mail
   d. Flyer or Announcement in Church Bulletin
   e. On the Webpage
   f. Social Media Groups (Facebook, Twitter, etc.)
   g. Other: _____

Section 2: Self-Assessment

In this section, statements are grouped into eight categories that correspond to the principles of CREATION Health – Choice, Rest, Environment, Activity, Trust in God, Interpersonal relationships, Outlook, and Nutrition. Congregation members are asked to respond by selecting which statement best applies to their situation: Almost Always, Sometimes, Rarely, or Never.

1. **Choice** – I am able to curb unhealthy habits and replace them with more beneficial alternatives.

2. **Rest** – Once a week, I take a day of rest in which I don't do my regular work and instead focus on rest, relationships, inspiration, and attitude.

3. **Environment** – I have added beautiful sights to my personal world. This may include plants, photographs, nature scenes, art, or other things that make me happy.

4. **Activity** – I get 30–60 minutes of exercise (such as walking, running, cycling, swimming, etc.) 3–6 days per week.

5. **Trust in God** – I talk honestly with God about my life, including my hopes, fears, desires, and needs. I believe God hears my prayers.

6. **Interpersonal Relationships** – I have friends I enjoy and with whom I can be myself. I share my true thoughts and feelings with at least one close friend.

7. **Outlook** – I accept myself despite my faults and limitations. I do not expect perfection in my life.

8. **Nutrition** – I avoid processed and fast food whenever possible.

Section 3: Areas of Interest

In this section, we ask congregation members to mark topics that they are interested in learning more about by participating in a program or class. Possible options include:

- Healthy Cooking
- Stress Management
- Divorce
- Prenatal Care
- Parenting Issues
- Caregiving and Aging Parents/ Relatives
- Midlife Changes
- Anger Management
- Depression

- Diabetes
- Self-Esteem
- Laughter, Humor, and Wellness
- Men's Health Issues
- Death and Dying
- Forgiveness
- Loss and Grief
- Prayer

RESOURCE D:

HEALTH MINISTRY LEADERSHIP MAP

Healthy 100 Church Ministry also developed an assessment based on CREATION Health that ministry leaders used to evaluate their existing activities, resources, and goals. This tool is divided into eight sections with thought-provoking questions intended to help start the conversation about what it would take to get a vibrant health ministry going.

- Section one addresses the congregation's understanding of whole-person health and the relationship of this understanding to the congregation's ministry philosophy.

- Section two focuses on the participation and support of church leaders for health ministry.

- Section three is about policies and practices related to CREATION Health and a vibrant health ministry.

- Section four helps ministry leaders assess the needs and opportunities that exist in their congregations and local communities.

- Section five addresses goals and objectives related to health ministry.

- Section six is about the congregation's health ministry programs and activities.

- Section seven focuses on the need for congregation leaders to be aware of, and to utilize, health and wellness resources in the congregation and community.

- Section eight moves things outward, with questions about the congregations' cooperation and collaboration with other agencies and the community.

This document has been revised since it was used in relation to the pilot program described in this report. To learn more about this resource, please contact Florida Hospital's Healthy 100 Church Ministry: http://www.healthy100churches.org/resources.[22]

RESOURCE E:

SAMPLE GOAL STATEMENTS

Defining expectations and setting goals early in the process of embarking on a Faith Community Nursing or health ministry journey is a critical step on the road to success. Good goal statements always include a clear time frame and a measureable result that you have determined will be the indicator of whether or not you have achieved success.

Example 1

Weak Goal Statement: We want members to learn how to prepare healthy foods by providing a cooking class.

Strong Goal Statement: Our goal is to teach members how to prepare healthy food by providing one healthy cooking class each month this year and sustaining an average attendance of at least 15 people per class.

Example 2

Weak Goal Statement: We want to demonstrate care for members of our congregation when they have overnight stays in the hospital.

Strong Goal Statement: Our goal is to demonstrate care for our congregants when they have overnight stays in the hospital by having a member of the health ministry team call or visit them within two hours of finding out about their hospitalization.

Example 3

Weak Goal Statement: We want to reduce the number of members in our congregation who have high blood pressure.

Strong Goal Statement: Our goal is to reduce the number of members in our congregation who have high blood pressure by 20 percent within the next six months. (Make sure to include an actual date of when the six months is up.)

RESOURCE F:

HELPFUL WEBSITES

The following websites provide useful information about Faith Community Nursing, Health Ministry Groups, Training, Fund-raising, and Foundations.

Church Health Center – www.parishnurses.org.

CREATION Health – www.CREATIONHealth.org.

Florida Hospital – www.FloridaHospital.org.

Health Ministries Association – www.hmassoc.org.

Healthy 100 – www.Healthy100.org.

Healthy 100 Church Ministry – www.Healthy100Churches.org.

Healthy People – www.HealthyPeople.gov.

International Faith Community Nursing –
http://churchhealthcenter.org/internationalfaithcommunitynursing.

Wheat Ridge Ministries – http://www.wheatridge.org/.

Winter Park Health Foundation – www.wphf.org.

ABOUT THE AUTHORS

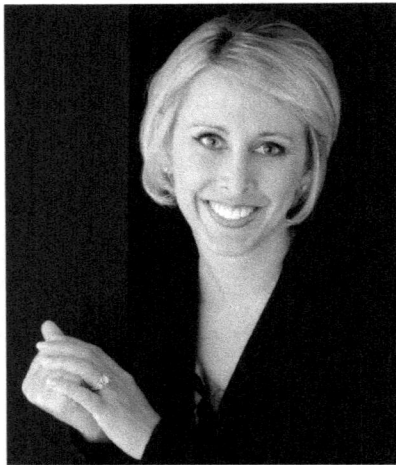

Stephanie Lind, MBA, is the Director of Healthy 100 Enterprise, contributing to Florida Hospital becoming a global leader in health and healing by empowering employees, the community, and the nation to live healthier, more fulfilling lives. In her previous role as Director for Healthy 100 Churches, she bridged hospitals and churches to create health ministries in one hundred eighty churches from twelve denominations. Lind received two undergraduate degrees from Union College and her MBA from Webster University. Her mission is to be a strategic, visionary leader by integrating wholistic health with business practices that bring significant and sustainable results. She is married to her treasured travel companion, Jeff Lind.

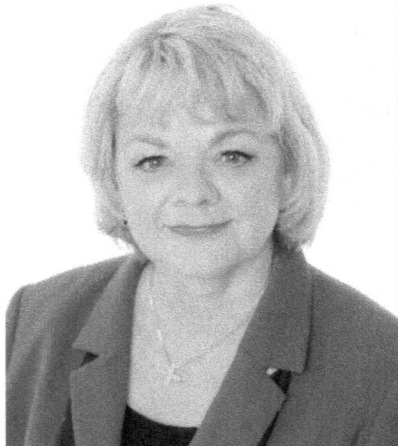

Dr. Susan K. Chase is a Professor and Associate Dean for Graduate Affairs in the College of Nursing at the University of Central Florida. She holds a doctorate in education from Harvard University, and has a master's in nursing education from New York University and bachelor's degrees from Columbia and Vanderbilt. She has served as a faith community nurse in Massachusetts and Florida and formerly taught at Boston College where she developed a joint master's degree in nursing and pastoral theology. She also taught at Florida Atlantic University and the University of Massachusetts, Worcester. She has published in the area of faith community nursing, end-of-life decision making, clinical judgment, and presence. She has published thirty articles in peer-reviewed journals, one book, and seventeen book chapters.

ACKNOWLEDGMENTS

Conducting a project of this scale, and then producing a report of this magnitude about it, would have been impossible without the support and wisdom of an entire team. We are deeply appreciative of the Winter Park Health Foundation for partnering with us to meet people where they are at – in congregations – and offer them a new resource for healthful living through Faith Community Nursing.

Rev. Jay Perez, vice president of mission and service excellence at Florida Hospital, played an instrumental role in casting a vision and helping us set goals.

Of course, none of this would have been possible without the enthusiastic participation of the five churches and their Faith Community Nurses: Regina Buchanan, Gigi Erwin, Denise Schmalzle, and Tonja Williams. Their commitment to improving the health of their communities was shown over and over again as they developed new methods of ministry to reach out to those who are hurting.

Our thanks also go to Candace Huber and Dr. Yvonne Seballo for serving as Faith Community Nurse Liaisons and providing inspiration and educational assistance to the project.

Todd Chobotar, Dr. David Biebel, and Rainey Turlington – thank you all for helping us create this report so that others can benefit from the lessons we learned on our journey with Faith Community Nursing.

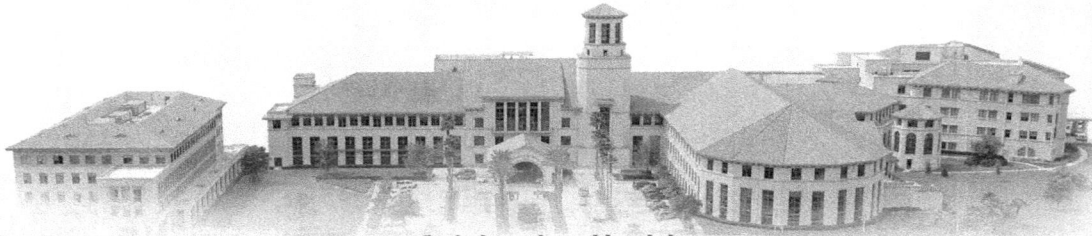

Celebration Health

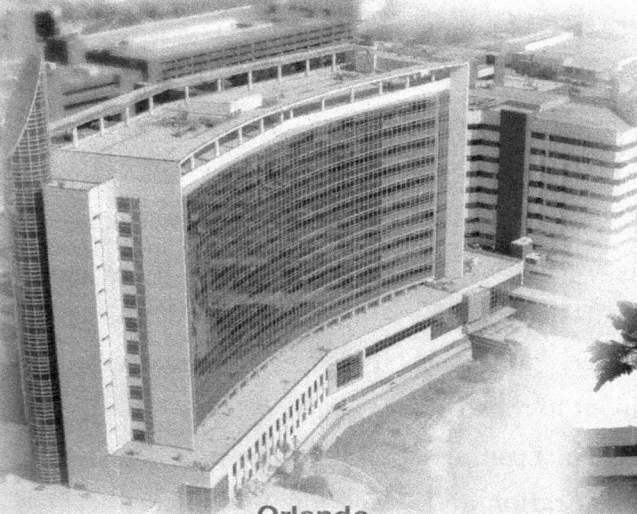

Orlando

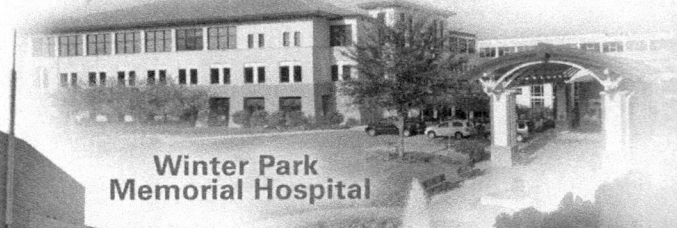

Winter Park Memorial Hospital

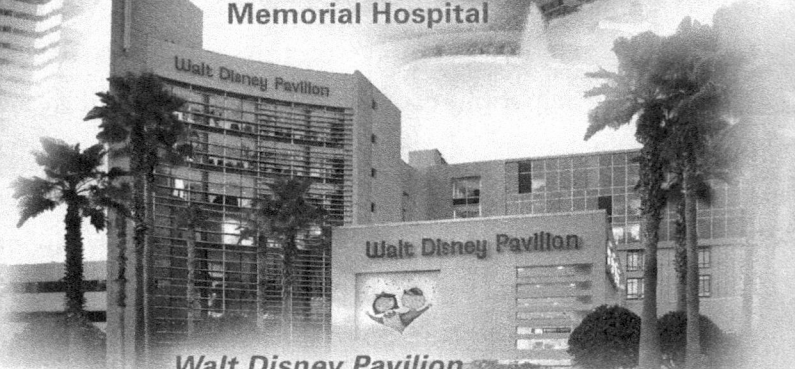

Walt Disney Pavilion
at Florida Hospital for Children

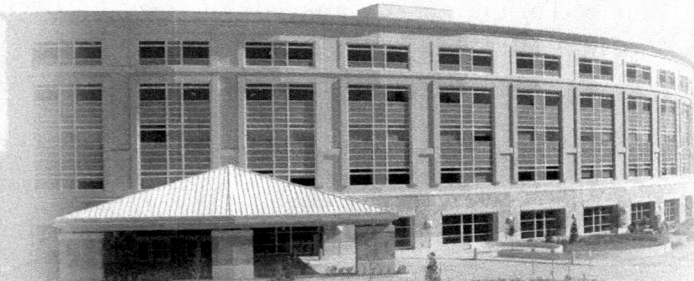

East Orlando

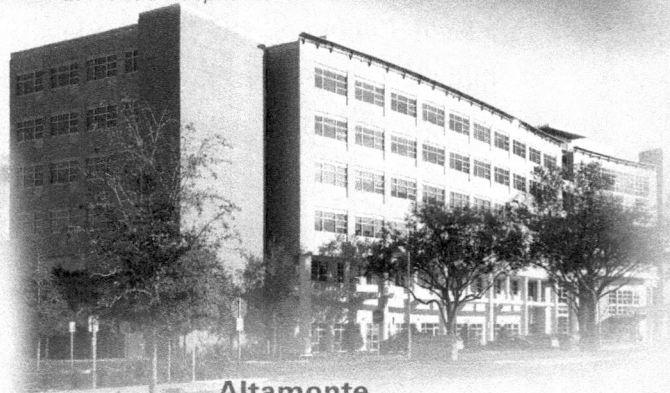

Altamonte

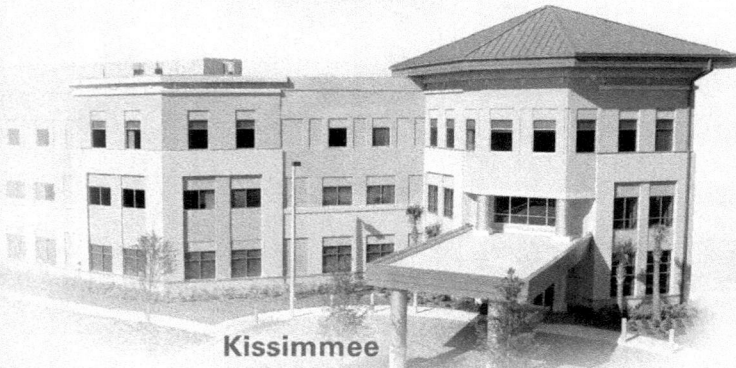

Kissimmee

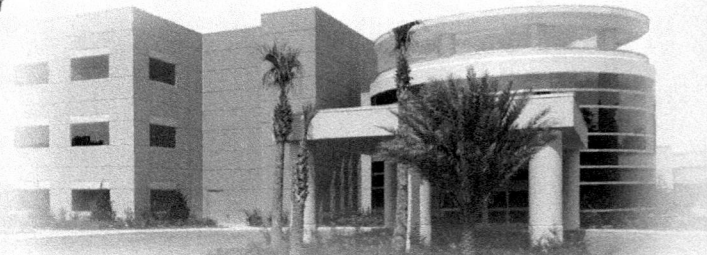

Apopka

FLORIDA HOSPITAL

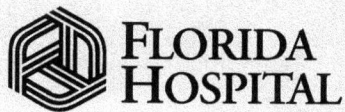

ABOUT THE PUBLISHER

For over one hundred years the mission of Florida Hospital has been: *To Extend the Healing Ministry of Christ*. Opened in 1908, Florida Hospital is comprised of eight hospital campuses housing over 2,400 beds and twenty-two walk-in medical centers. With over 19,000 employees – including 2,200 doctors and 6,600 nurses – Florida Hospital serves the residents and guests of Orlando, the No. 1 tourist destination in the world. Florida Hospital has over 1.7 million patient visits a year. Florida Hospital is a Christian, faith-based hospital that believes in providing whole-person care to all patients – mind, body, and spirit. Hospital fast facts include:

LARGEST ADMITTING HOSPITAL IN AMERICA – Ranked No. 1 in the nation for inpatient admissions by the *American Hospital Association*.

AMERICA'S HEART HOSPITAL – Ranked No. 1 in the nation for number of heart procedures performed each year, averaging 22,000 cases annually. MSNBC named Florida Hospital "America's Heart Hospital" for being the No. 1 hospital fighting America's No. 1 killer – heart disease.

HOSPITAL OF THE FUTURE – At the turn of the century, the *Wall Street Journal* named Florida Hospital the "Hospital of the Future."

ONE OF AMERICA'S BEST HOSPITALS – Recognized by *U.S. News & World Report* as "One of America's Best Hospitals" for ten years. Clinical specialties recognized have included: Cardiology, Orthopaedics, Neurology & Neurosurgery, Urology, Gynecology, Digestive Disorders, Hormonal Disorders, Kidney Disease, Ear, Nose & Throat, and Endocrinology.

LEADER IN SENIOR CARE – Florida Hospital serves the largest number of seniors in America through Medicare with a goal for each patient to experience a "Century of Health" by living to a healthy hundred.

TOP BIRTHING CENTER – *Fit Pregnancy* magazine named Florida Hospital one of the "Top 10 Best Places in the Country to have a Baby." As a result, *The Discovery Health Channel* struck a three-year production deal with Florida Hospital to host a live broadcast called "Birth Day Live." Florida Hospital annually delivers over 10,000 babies.

CORPORATE ALLIANCES – Florida Hospital maintains corporate alliance relationships with a select group of Fortune 500 companies including Disney, Nike, Johnson & Johnson, Philips, AGFA, and Stryker.

DISNEY PARTNERSHIP – Florida Hospital is the Central Florida health & wellness resource of the *Walt Disney World*® Resort. Florida Hospital also partnered with Disney to build the groundbreaking health and wellness facility called Florida Hospital Celebration Health located in Disney's town of Celebration, Florida. Disney and Florida Hospital recently partnered to build a new state-of-the-art Children's Hospital.

HOSPITAL OF THE 21ST CENTURY – Florida Hospital Celebration Health was awarded the *Premier Patient Services Innovator Award* as "The Model for Healthcare Delivery in the 21st Century."

SPORTS EXPERTS – Florida Hospital is the official hospital of the Orlando *Magic* NBA basketball team. In addition, Florida Hospital has an enduring track record of providing exclusive medical care to many sports organizations. These organizations have included: Disney's Wide World of Sports, Walt Disney World's Marathon Weekend, the Capital One Bowl, and University of Central Florida Athletics. Florida Hospital has also provided comprehensive healthcare services for the World Cup and Olympics.

PRINT RECOGNITION – *Self* magazine named Florida Hospital one of America's "Top 10 Hospitals for Women." *Modern Healthcare* magazine proclaimed it one of America's best hospitals for cardiac care.

CONSUMER CHOICE AWARD WINNER – Florida Hospital has received the *Consumer Choice Award* from the National Research Corporation every year from 1996 to the present.

FLORIDA HOSPITAL | 601 E. Rollins Street, Orlando, FL 32803 | www.FloridaHospital.org | 407-303-5600

CREATION HEALTH | LIVE LIFE TO THE FULLEST

NOTES

1   Source: "Doctors Perform Thousands of Unnecessary Surgeries" (June 20, 2013). Posted online at: http://www.usatoday.com/story/news/nation/2013/06/18/unnecessary-surgery-usa-today-investigation/2435009/.

2   Source: "Chronic Diseases: The Leading Causes of Death and Disability in the United States" (May 9, 2014). Posted online at: http://www.cdc.gov/chronicdisease/overview/index.htm?s_cid=ostltsdyk_govd_203.

3   Katherine Harmon, "Prescription Drug Deaths Increase Dramatically," *Scientific American*, April 6, 2010. Posted online at: http://www.scientificamerican.com/article/prescription-drug-deaths/.

4   "Retail Prescription Drugs Filled at Pharmacies (Annual per Capita by Age)," *The Henry J. Kaiser Family Foundation*, accessed June 3, 2014. Posted online at: http://kff.org/other/state-indicator/retail-rx-drugs-by-age/.

5   See Gary B. Ferngren *Medicine and Healthcare in Early Christianity* (Baltimore, MD: 2009).

6   Phyllis Ann Solari-Twadell (ed.) and Mary Ann McDermott (ed.) *Faith Community Nursing: Promoting Whole Person Health within Faith Communities* (Thousand Oaks, CA: Sage Publications, 1999), 3.

7   Curriculum guidance for training Faith Community Nurses (also known as "Parish Nurses") is available through the International Faith Community Nurse Resource Center: https://www.facebook.com/pages/International-Parish-Nurse-Resource-Center-IPNRC/193648440675125.

8   Amy Frykholm, "Fit for Ministry," *Christian Century*, Oct. 22, 2012. Posted online at: http://www.christiancentury.org/article/2012-10/fit-ministry.

9   "Clergy Members Suffer From Burnout, Poor Health." Posted online at: http://www.npr.org/templates/story/story.php?storyId=128957149.

10   *Pastoral Health Assessment October 2010* (Lutheran Church Missouri Synod: Austin, TX, 2010), 8. PDF of this report is posted online at: http://txdistlcms.org/downloads/Pastoral_Health_Assessment_Texas_2010.pdf.

11   See "Clergy Health: Who Cares for the Caregivers?" *Duke Today* (June 28, 2012). Posted online at: http://today.duke.edu/2012/06/clergyhealth.

12 Kate Santich, "Growing Number of Churches Hiring Nurses to Motivate the Faithful," *Orlando Sentinel* (July 2, 2011). Posted online at: http://www.orlandosentinel.com/health/os-nurses-in-churches-20110702_1_nurses-faith-community-congregations.

13 "Churches Hiring Nurses to Promote Wellness," *Church Leaders*. Posted online at: http://www.churchleaders.com/pastors/pastor-articles/152491-churches-hiring-nurses-to-promote-wellness.html.

14 Kimberly Lord Stewart, "First Lady Michelle Obama Announces Winners of Let's Move! Video Challenge," *Examiner.com*. Posted online at: http://www.examiner.com/article/first-lady-michelle-obama-announces-winners-of-let-s-move-video-challenge.

15 For information on the Florida Hospital Celebration Health Assessment, see: http://www.celebrationhealthassessment.com/.

16 This summary of findings is based on information provided by Susan K. Chase, EdD, project evaluator.

17 Note that as this paper goes to press, the program and name of Florida Hospital's effort to support health ministry in churches is in transition. Updates may be found at: http://www.healthy100churches.org/. The focus of this report is the three-year pilot evaluation that was conducted as a result of a grant from the Winter Park Health Foundation. Nothing about further developments of this or similar efforts of Florida Hospital should be inferred from this report.

18 SF-12® is a registered trademark of Medical Outcomes Trust© 1994, 2002 by QualityMetric Incorporated and Medical Outcomes Trust. All rights reserved.

19 The Spiritual Well-Being Scale, developed by Dr. Craig W. Ellison and Dr. Raymond F. Paloutzian, provides an overall measure of the perception of spiritual quality of life, as well as subscale scores for Religious and Existential Well-Being. For information on this instrument, view: http://www.lifeadvance.com/spiritual-well-being-scale.html.

20 For information on Health Ministries Association, see: https://hmassoc.org/. For information about the International Faith Community Nurse Resource Center, see: https://www.facebook.com/pages/International-Parish-Nurse-Resource-Center-IPNRC/193648440675125.

21 For information regarding this and other Healthy 100 Churches resources, visit: http://www.healthy100churches.org/resources.

22 A similar resource is available for download at: http://www.wheatridge.org/download-the-self-study.

LEAD YOUR COMMUNITY
TO HEALTHY
LIVING

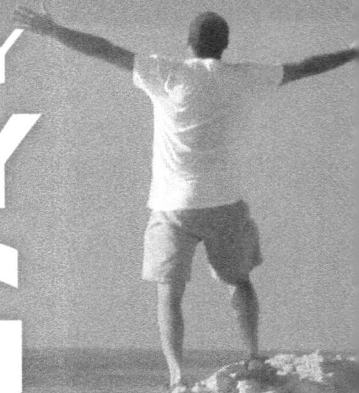

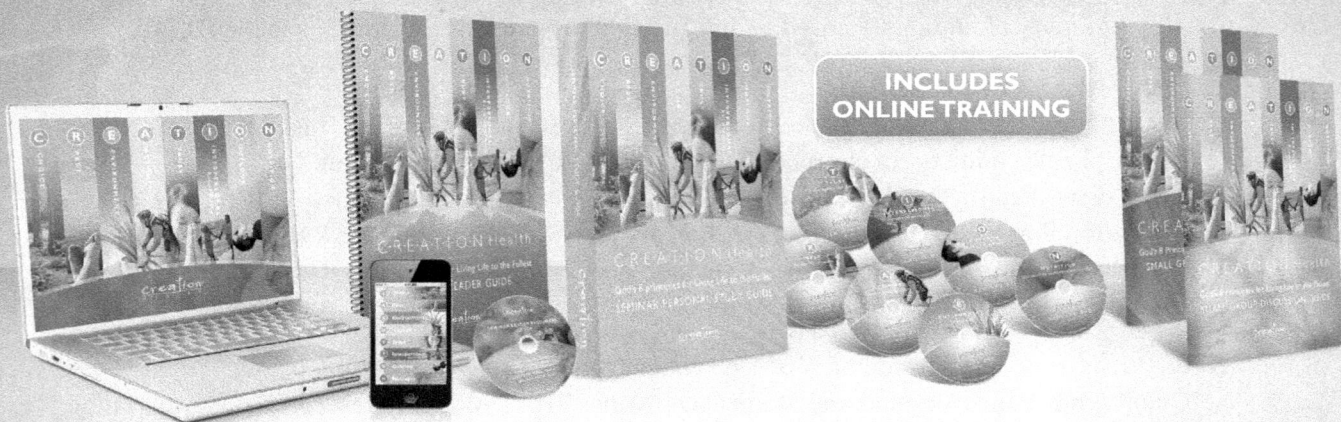

Seminar Leader Kit
Everything a leader needs to conduct this seminar successfully, including key questions to facilitate group discussion and PowerPoint™ presentations for each of the eight principles.

Participant Guide
A study guide with essential information from each of the eight lessons along with outlines, self assessments, and questions for people to fill in as they follow along.

Small Group Kit
It's easy to lead a small group using the CREATION Health videos, the Small Group Leaders Guide, and the Small Group Discussion Guide.

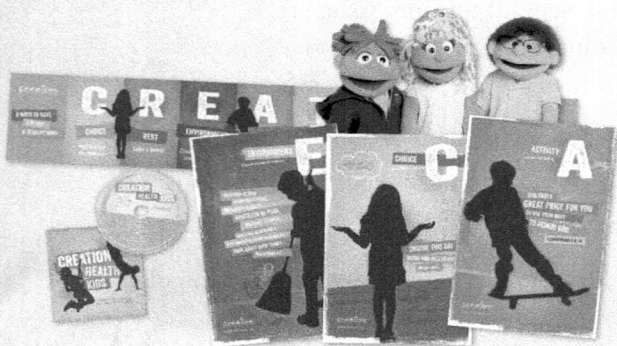

CREATION Kids
CREATION Health Kids can make a big difference in homes, schools, and congregations. Lead kids in your community to healthier, happier living.

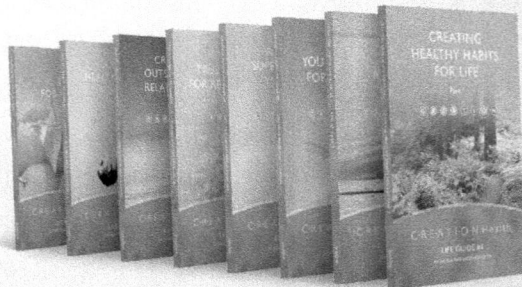

Life Guide Series
These guides include questions designed to help individuals or small groups study the depths of every principle and learn strategies for integrating them into everyday life.

GUIDES AND ASSESSMENTS

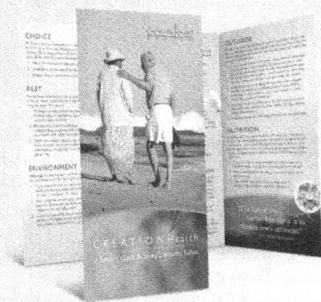

Pregnancy Guides
Expert advice on how to be CREATION Healthy while expecting.

Senior Guide
Share the CREATION Health principles with seniors and help them be healthier and happier as they live life to the fullest.

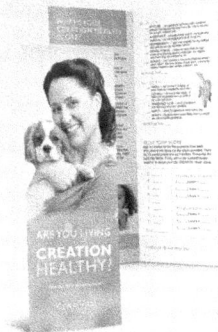

Self-Assessment
This instrument raises awareness about how CREATION Healthy a person is in each of the eight major areas of wellness.

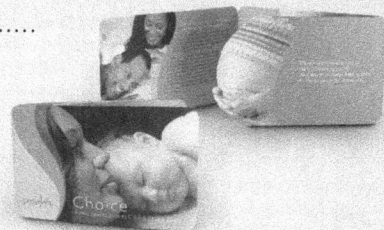

Pocket Guide
A tool for keeping people committed to living all of the CREATION Health principles daily.

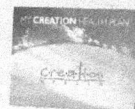

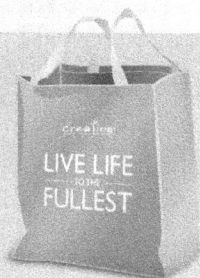

Tote Bag
A convenient way for bringing CREATION Health materials to and from class.

MARKETING MATERIALS

Postcards, Posters, Stationery, and more
You can effectively advertise and generate community excitement about your CREATION Health seminar with a wide range of available marketing materials such as enticing postcards, flyers, posters, and more.

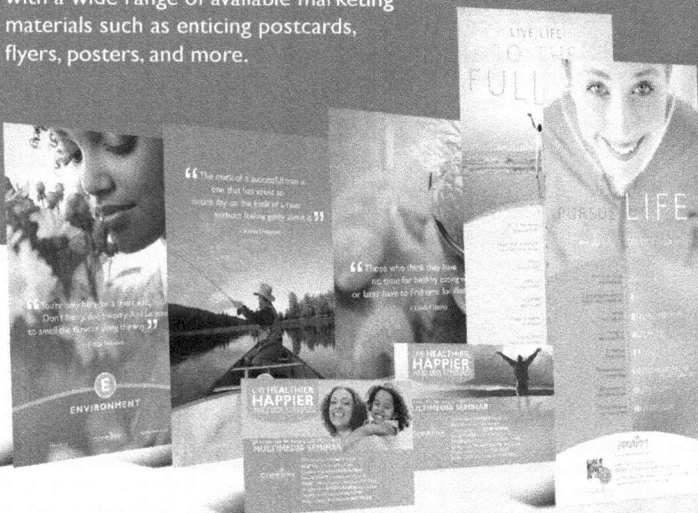

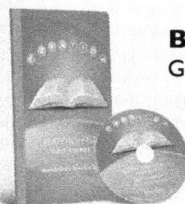

Tumbler
Practice good Nutrition and keep yourself hydrated with a CREATION Health tumbler in an assortment of fun colors.

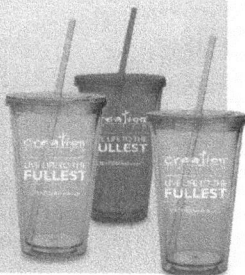

Bible Stories
God is interested in our physical, mental and spiritual well-being. Throughout the Bible you can discover the eight principles for full life.

CREATION HEALTH BOOKS

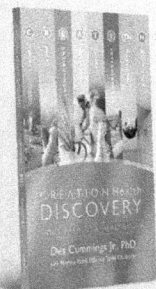

CREATION Health Discovery
Written by Des Cummings Jr., PhD, Monica Reed, MD, and Todd Chobotar, this wonderful companion resource introduces people to the CREATION Health philosophy and lifestyle.

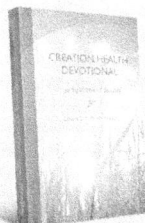

CREATION Health Devotional
(English: Hardcover / Spanish: Softcover)
In this devotional you will discover stories about experiencing God's grace in the tough times, God's delight in triumphant times, and God's presence in peaceful times.

CREATION HEALTH RESOURCES

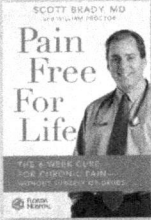

Pain Free For Life (Hardcover)
In *Pain Free For Life*, Scott C. Brady, MD – founder of Florida Hospital's Brady Institute for Health – shares for the first time with the general public his dramatically successful solution for chronic back pain, fibromyalgia, chronic headaches, irritable bowel syndrome, and other "impossible to cure" pains. Dr. Brady leads pain-racked readers to a pain-free life using powerful mind-body-spirit strategies used at the Brady Institute – where more than 80 percent of his chronic-pain patients have achieved 80–100 percent pain relief within weeks.

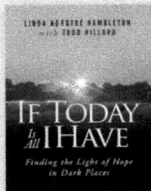

If Today Is All I Have (Softcover)
At its heart, Linda's captivating account chronicles the struggle to reconcile her three dreams of experiencing life as a "normal woman" with the tough realities of her medical condition. Her journey is punctuated with insights that are at times humorous, painful, provocative, and life-affirming.

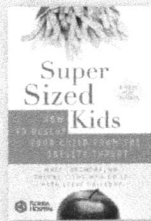

SuperSized Kids (Hardcover)
In *SuperSized Kids*, Walt Larimore, MD, and Sherri Flynt, MPH, RD, LD, show how the mushrooming childhood obesity epidemic is destroying children's lives, draining family resources, and pushing America dangerously close to a total healthcare collapse – while also explaining, step by step, how parents can work to avert the coming crisis by taking control of the weight challenges facing every member of their family.

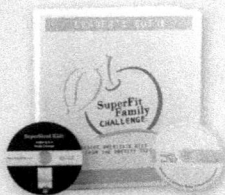

SuperFit Family Challenge – Leader's Guide
Perfect for your community, church, small group or other settings.
The SuperFit Family Challenge Leader's Guide Includes:

- 8 Weeks of pre-designed PowerPoint™ presentations.

- Professionally designed marketing materials and group handouts from direct mailers to reading guides.

- Training directly from Author Sherri Flynt, MPH, RD, LD, across 6 audio CDs.

- Media coverage and FAQ on DVD.

CREATION HEALTH RESOURCES

Forgive To Live (English: Hardcover / Spanish: Softcover)
In *Forgive to Live* Dr. Tibbits presents the scientifically proven steps for forgiveness –taken from the first clinical study of its kind conducted by Stanford University and Florida Hospital.

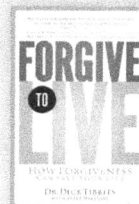

Forgive To Live Workbook (Softcover)
This interactive guide will show you how to forgive – insight by insight, step by step – in a workable plan that can effectively reduce your anger, improve your health, and put you in charge of your life again, no matter how deep your hurts.

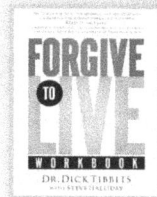

Forgive To Live Devotional (Hardcover)
In his powerful new devotional Dr. Dick Tibbits reveals the secret to forgiveness. This compassionate devotional is a stirring look at the true meaning of forgiveness. Each of the 56 spiritual insights includes motivational Scripture, an inspirational prayer, and two thought-provoking questions. The insights are designed to encourage your journey as you begin to *Forgive to Live*.

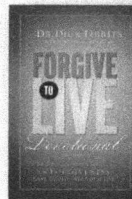

Forgive To Live God's Way (Softcover)
Forgiveness is so important that our very lives depend on it. Churches teach us that we should forgive, but how do you actually learn to forgive? In this spiritual workbook noted author, psychologist, and ordained minister Dr. Dick Tibbits takes you step-by-step through an eight-week forgiveness format that is easy to understand and follow.

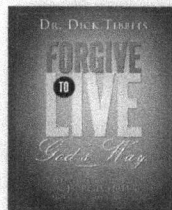

Forgive To Live Leader's Guide
Perfect for your community, church, small group or other settings.
The Forgive to Live Leader's Guide Includes:

- 8 Weeks of pre-designed PowerPoint™ presentations.

- Professionally designed customizable marketing materials and group handouts on CD-Rom.

- Training directly from author of *Forgive to Live* Dr. Dick Tibbits across 6 audio CDs.

- Media coverage DVD.

- CD-Rom containing all files in digital format for easy home or professional printing.

- A copy of the first study of its kind conducted by Stanford University and Florida Hospital showing a link between decreased blood pressure and forgiveness.

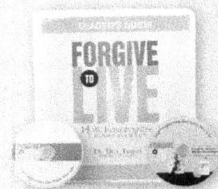

CREATION HEALTH RESOURCES

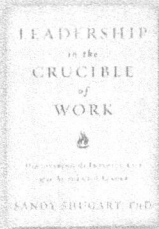

Leadership in the Crucible of Work (Hardcover)
What is the first and most important work of a leader? (The answer may surprise you.) In *Leadership in the Crucible of Work*, noted speaker, poet, and college president Dr. Sandy Shugart takes readers on an unforgettable journey to the heart of what it means to become an authentic leader.

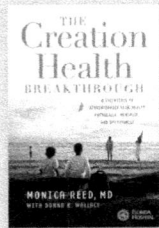

CREATION Health Breakthrough (Hardcover)
Blending science and lifestyle recommendations, Monica Reed, MD, prescribes eight essentials that will help reverse harmful health habits and prevent disease. Discover how intentional choices, rest, environment, activity, trust, relationships, outlook, and nutrition can put a person on the road to wellness. Features a three-day total body rejuvenation therapy and four-phase life transformation plan.

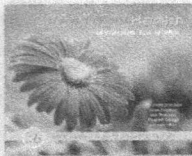

CREATION Health Devotional for Women (English)
Written for women by women, the *CREATION Health Devotional for Women* is based on the principles of whole-person wellness represented in CREATION Health. Spirits will be lifted and lives rejuvenated by the message of each unique chapter. This book is ideal for women's prayer groups, to give as a gift, or just to buy for your own edification and encouragement.

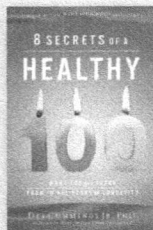

8 Secrets of a Healthy 100 (Softcover)
Can you imagine living to a Healthy 100 years of age? Dr. Des Cummings Jr., explores the principles practiced by the "All-stars of Longevity" to live longer and more abundantly. Take a journey through the 8 Secrets and you will be inspired to imagine living to a Healthy 100.

Florida Hospital Publishing presents the *Healthcare & Leadership* monograph series.

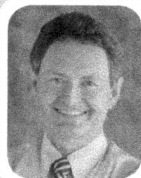

Building Bridges: A Guide to Optimizing Physician-Hospital Relationships, written by Dr. Ted Hamilton. In these pages you will find help not only in relating more effectively to physicians, but in developing initiatives that will build healthier relationships between hospitals and medical staff that will ultimately improve patient care. A valuable publication for leadership of mission-focused health care organizations and their physician partners.

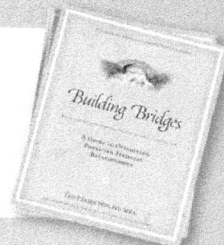

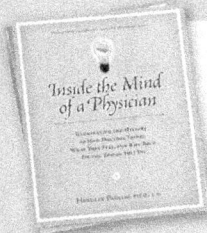

Inside the Mind of a Physician, written by Dr. Herdley Paolini, does a great service by opening the inner world of physicians and helping us understand them, how to relate to them, and how to support them in their critical role in health care. Her insights will be of great value to everyone from hospital administrators and clinical staff, to insurance providers, government agencies, and anyone who interacts with physicians.

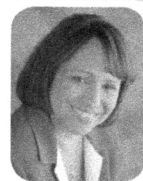

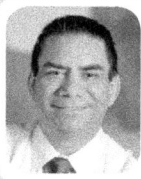

The Patient Experience, written by Jay Perez, offers simple solutions that everyone can do to create an exceptional patient experience. Hospitals are so clinically oriented they often overlook the emotional and relational aspects of patient care, which is how many patients judge their experience. When caregivers let patients know who they are, what they do, and why the care it creates a great sense of hope, trust, and belonging.

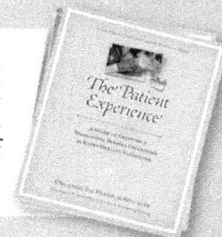

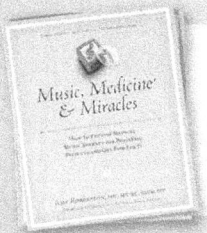

Music, Medicine & Miracles: How to Provide Medical Music Therapy for Pediatric Patients and Get Paid for It, written by Amy Robertson, founder of the Music Therapy program at *Florida Hospital for Children*, offers in-depth solutions for utilizing music to help pediatric patients heal in mind, body and spirit. Music Therapy is becoming an important part of the mission of many health care facilities.

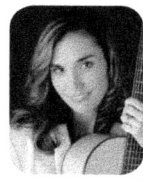

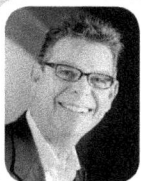

Making History Together: How to Create Innovate Strategic Alliances to Fuel the Growth of Your Company, written by Keith Lowe, takes you through the steps of how Florida Hospital creates and cultivates outstanding strategic alliance relationships—and how you can, too. ***Have you ever wondered*** how Florida Hospital creates world-class partnerships with companies like Disney, Nike, GE, IBM, Philips, Johnson & Johnson, and Bayer? Now you can discover the secrets for yourself.

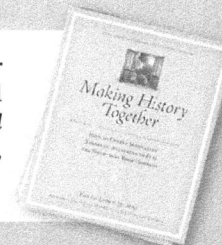

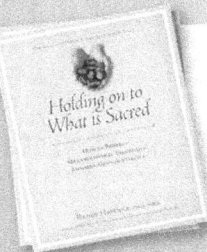

Holding on to What is Sacred, written by Dr. Randy Haffner, lays out a persuasive vision for how organizations can stay focused on their true values. The most intriguing aspect of the monograph is Dr. Haffner's concept of Confessional Identity. It seeks the spiritual heart of an organization's reason for being. Why? Because so much is at stake. Your employees need to know why you exist and why their efforts matter. Your customers need to know why you really care. Your leaders need to embrace your core convictions wholeheartedly or they will lose direction.

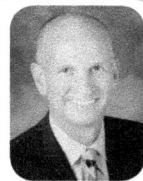

The *Florida Hospital Healthcare and Leadership Monograph* series are perfect for:
Hospitals | Clinicians | Music Therapists | Business Professionals | Chaplains | And many more!

FLORIDA HOSPITAL
The skill to heal. The spirit to care.

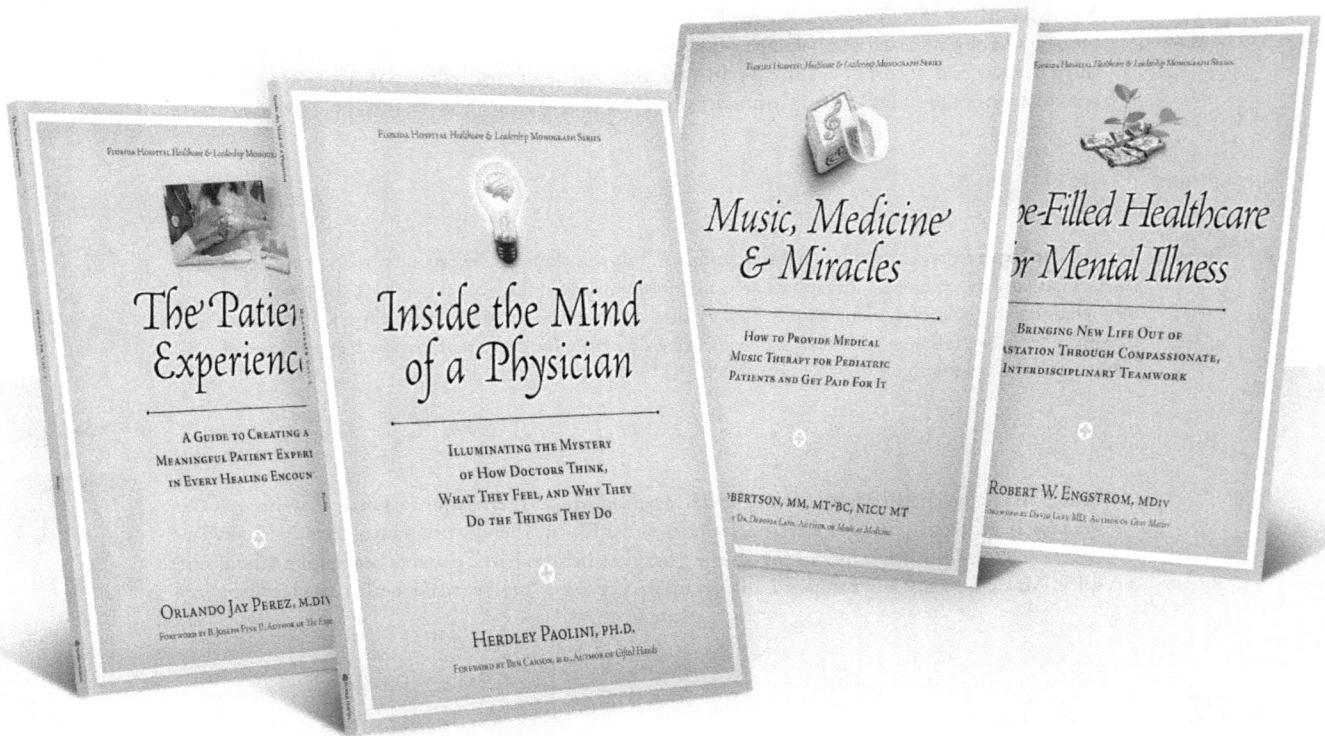

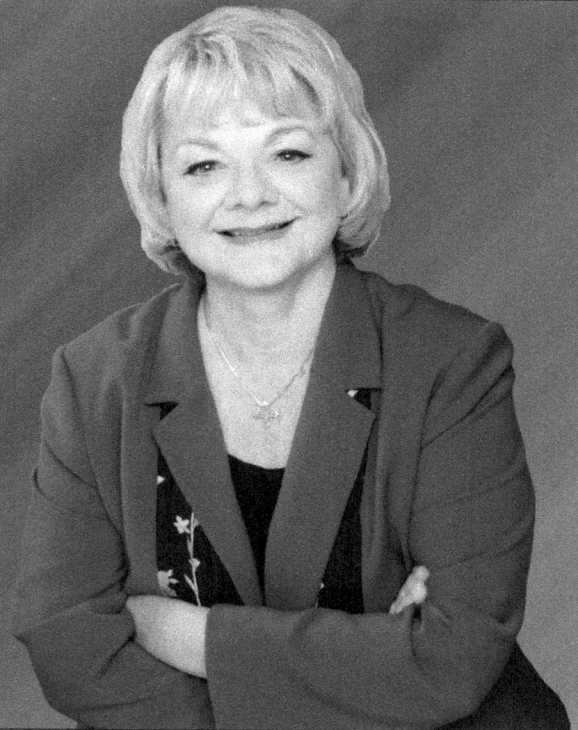

HEAR MORE FROM STEPHANIE LIND

Let Stephanie Lind guide your team through the steps to significant and sustainable results.

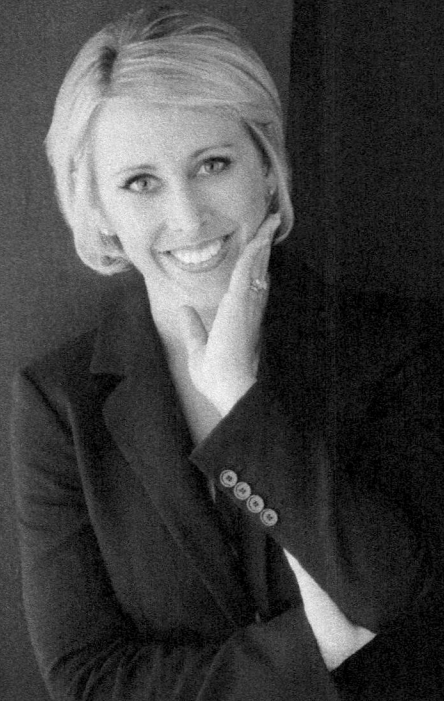

STEPHANIE LIND'S TOPICS:

+ CREATION Health Philosophy: "Living Life to the Fullest"

+ Bridging Hospital & Church Relationships

+ Nonprofit Sustainability: When it's essential to connect money and mission

SPEAKING/CONSULTING – Have topic you'd like to hear Stephanie speak on that's not listed here? Simply fill out one of our Speaker Inquiry forms at FloridaHospitalPublishing.com, and we will work with you to customize a presentation that is just right for your group. Or inquire about Stephanie's consulting availability to work directly with your leadership team.

OTHER SPEAKERS – Need to schedule a speaker for your next conference, seminar or event? Florida Hospital Speakers Bureau can provide exactly what you need. Whether it's a keynote, a daylong presentation, or a speech catered to your needs, we have a growing list of speakers dedicated to bringing you the most up-to-date in Whole Person Health information.

To book a speaker or register for a seminar, visit

www.FloridaHospitalPublishing.com

www.ingramcontent.com/pod-product-compliance
Lightning Source LLC
Chambersburg PA
CBHW081650270326
41933CB00018B/3414